ASSESSING AND IMPROVING

VALUE

IN CANCER CARE

Workshop Summ~

D1298227

Adam Schickedanz, *Rapporteur*

National Cancer Policy Forum
Board on Health Care Services

INSTITUTE OF MEDICINE
OF THE NATIONAL ACADEMIES

THE NATIONAL ACADEMIES PRESS
Washington, D.C.
www.nap.edu

THE NATIONAL ACADEMIES PRESS   500 Fifth Street, N.W.   Washington, DC 20001

NOTICE: The project that is the subject of this report was approved by the Governing Board of the National Research Council, whose members are drawn from the councils of the National Academy of Sciences, the National Academy of Engineering, and the Institute of Medicine.

This study was supported by Contract Nos. HHSN261200611002C, 200-2005-13434 TO #1, and 223-01-2460 to #27, between the National Academy of Sciences and the National Cancer Institute, the Centers for Disease Control and Prevention, and the Food and Drug Administration, respectively. This study was also supported by the American Cancer Society, the American Society of Clinical Oncology, the Association of American Cancer Institutes, and C-Change. Any opinions, findings, conclusions, or recommendations expressed in this publication are those of the author(s) and do not necessarily reflect the view of the organizations or agencies that provided support for this project.

International Standard Book Number-13: 978-0-309-13814-7
International Standard Book Number-10: 0-309-13814-0

Additional copies of this report are available from the National Academies Press, 500 Fifth Street, N.W., Lockbox 285, Washington, DC, 20055; (800) 624-6242 or (202) 334-3313 (in the Washington metropolitan area); Internet, http://www.nap.edu.

For more information about the Institute of Medicine, visit the IOM home page at **www.iom.edu**.

Printed in the United States of America

The serpent has been a symbol of long life, healing, and knowledge among almost all cultures and religions since the beginning of recorded history. The serpent adopted as a logotype by the Institute of Medicine is a relief carving from ancient Greece, now held by the Staatliche Museen in Berlin.

Suggested citation: IOM (Institute of Medicine). 2009. *Assessing and improving value in cancer care: Workshop summary.* Washington, DC: The National Academies Press.

*"Knowing is not enough; we must apply.
Willing is not enough; we must do."*
—Goethe

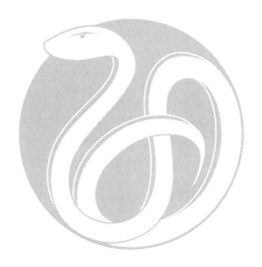

INSTITUTE OF MEDICINE
OF THE NATIONAL ACADEMIES

Advising the Nation. Improving Health.

THE NATIONAL ACADEMIES
Advisers to the Nation on Science, Engineering, and Medicine

The **National Academy of Sciences** is a private, nonprofit, self-perpetuating society of distinguished scholars engaged in scientific and engineering research, dedicated to the furtherance of science and technology and to their use for the general welfare. Upon the authority of the charter granted to it by the Congress in 1863, the Academy has a mandate that requires it to advise the federal government on scientific and technical matters. Dr. Ralph J. Cicerone is president of the National Academy of Sciences.

The **National Academy of Engineering** was established in 1964, under the charter of the National Academy of Sciences, as a parallel organization of outstanding engineers. It is autonomous in its administration and in the selection of its members, sharing with the National Academy of Sciences the responsibility for advising the federal government. The National Academy of Engineering also sponsors engineering programs aimed at meeting national needs, encourages education and research, and recognizes the superior achievements of engineers. Dr. Charles M. Vest is president of the National Academy of Engineering.

The **Institute of Medicine** was established in 1970 by the National Academy of Sciences to secure the services of eminent members of appropriate professions in the examination of policy matters pertaining to the health of the public. The Institute acts under the responsibility given to the National Academy of Sciences by its congressional charter to be an adviser to the federal government and, upon its own initiative, to identify issues of medical care, research, and education. Dr. Harvey V. Fineberg is president of the Institute of Medicine.

The **National Research Council** was organized by the National Academy of Sciences in 1916 to associate the broad community of science and technology with the Academy's purposes of furthering knowledge and advising the federal government. Functioning in accordance with general policies determined by the Academy, the Council has become the principal operating agency of both the National Academy of Sciences and the National Academy of Engineering in providing services to the government, the public, and the scientific and engineering communities. The Council is administered jointly by both Academies and the Institute of Medicine. Dr. Ralph J. Cicerone and Dr. Charles M. Vest are chair and vice chair, respectively, of the National Research Council.

www.national-academies.org

PLANNING COMMITTEE ON ASSESSING AND IMPROVING VALUE IN CANCER CARE

SCOTT D. RAMSEY (*Chair*), Full Member, Fred Hutchinson Cancer Research Center

PETER BACH, Associate Member, Memorial Sloan-Kettering Cancer Center

THOMAS BURISH, Past Chair, American Cancer Society Board, and Provost, Notre Dame University

ROBERT L. ERWIN, President, Marti Nelson Cancer Foundation

BETTY FERRELL, Research Scientist, City of Hope National Medical Center

PATRICIA GANZ, Director, Division of Cancer Prevention and Control Research, Jonsson Comprehensive Cancer Center, UCLA

ALLEN LICHTER, Executive Vice President and Chief Executive Officer, American Society of Clinical Oncology

HAROLD L. MOSES, Director Emeritus, Vanderbilt-Ingram Cancer Center

SEAN TUNIS, Founder and Director, Center for Medical Technology Policy

Project Staff

ROGER HERDMAN, Project Director, National Cancer Policy Forum and Board on Health Care Services

ADAM SCHICKEDANZ, Christine Mirzayan Science and Technology Policy Graduate Fellow

MICHAEL PARK, Senior Program Assistant

ASHLEY McWILLIAMS, Senior Program Assistant

LAURA LEVIT, Program Officer

CHRISTINE MICHEEL, Program Officer

NATIONAL CANCER POLICY FORUM[1]

HAROLD MOSES (*Chair*), Director Emeritus, Vanderbilt-Ingram Cancer Center
FRED APPELBAUM, Director, Clinical Research Division, Fred Hutchinson Cancer Research Center
PETER BACH, Associate Attending Physician, Memorial Sloan-Kettering Cancer Center
EDWARD BENZ, JR., President, Dana Farber Cancer Institute and Director, Harvard Cancer Center
THOMAS BURISH, Past Chair, American Cancer Society Board of Directors and Provost, Notre Dame University
MICHAELE CHAMBLEE CHRISTIAN, Division of Cancer Treatment and Diagnosis, National Cancer Institute
ROBERT ERWIN, President, Marti Nelson Cancer Foundation
BETTY FERRELL, Research Scientist, City of Hope National Medical Center
JOSEPH FRAUMENI, JR., Director, Division of Cancer Epidemiology and Genetics, National Cancer Institute
PATRICIA GANZ, Professor, UCLA Schools of Medicine & Public Health, Jonsson Comprehensive Cancer Center
ROBERT GERMAN, Associate Director for Science, Division of Cancer Prevention and Control, Centers for Disease Control and Prevention
ROY HERBST, Chief, Thoracic/Head & Neck Medical Oncology, M.D. Anderson Cancer Center
THOMAS KEAN, Executive Director, C-Change
JOHN MENDELSOHN, President, M.D. Anderson Cancer Center
JOHN NIEDERHUBER, Director, National Cancer Institute

---

[1] Institute of Medicine forums and roundtables do not issue, review, or approve individual documents. The responsibility for the published workshop summary rests with the workshop rapporteurs and the institution. The Institute of Medicine (IOM) established the National Cancer Policy Forum (NCPF), effective on May 1, 2005, to succeed the National Cancer Policy Board (NCPB), which existed from 1996 to 2005. IOM forums are designed to allow government, industry, academic, and other representatives to meet and confer privately on subject areas of mutual interest. NCPF is the successor to the NCPB in providing a focus within the National Academies for the consideration of issues in science, clinical medicine, public health, and public policy relevant to the goals of preventing, palliating, and curing cancer.

DAVID PARKINSON, President and CEO, Oncology Research and Development, Nodality, Inc.

SCOTT RAMSEY, Full Member, Cancer Prevention Program, Division of Public Health Science, Fred Hutchinson Cancer Research Center

JOHN WAGNER, Full Member, Executive Director, Clinical Pharmacology, Merck and Company, Inc.

JANET WOODCOCK, Deputy Commissioner and Chief Medical Officer, Food and Drug Administration

Staff

ROGER HERDMAN, Director, National Cancer Policy Forum and Board on Health Care Services

ERIN BALOGH, Research Associate

LAURA LEVIT, Program Officer

ASHLEY McWILLIAMS, Senior Program Assistant

CHRISTINE MICHEEL, Program Officer

SHARYL NASS, Senior Program Officer

MICHAEL PARK, Senior Program Assistant

ADAM SCHICKEDANZ, Christine Mirzayan Science and Technology Policy Graduate Fellow

ANIA WOLOSZYNSKA-READ, Christine Mirzayan Science and Technology Policy Graduate Fellow

Reviewers

This report has been reviewed in draft form by individuals chosen for their diverse perspectives and technical expertise, in accordance with procedures approved by the National Research Council's Report Review Committee. The purpose of this independent review is to provide candid and critical comments that will assist the institution in making its published report as sound as possible and to ensure that the report meets institutional standards for objectivity, evidence, and responsiveness to the study charge. The review comments and draft manuscript remain confidential to protect the integrity of the process. We wish to thank the following individuals for their review of this report:

CRAIG EARLE, Cancer Care Ontario and Ontario Institute for Cancer Research

PATRICIA GANZ, UCLA Schools of Medicine & Public Health, Jonsson Comprehensive Cancer Center

ALLEN LICHTER, American Society of Clinical Oncology

STEVE PHURROUGH, Center for Medicare and Medicaid Services

Although the reviewers listed above have provided many constructive comments and suggestions, they were not asked to endorse the final draft of the report before its release. The review of this report was overseen by

Sharon Murphy. Appointed by the Institute of Medicine, she was responsible for making certain that an independent examination of this report was carried out in accordance with institutional procedures and that all review comments were carefully considered. Responsibility for the final content of this report rests entirely with the rapporteur and the institution.

Contents

Preface

Oncology is similar to the other areas in health care in that it is under pressure to control expenditures while maintaining or improving quality of care and patient outcomes such that the value of oncology care is enhanced. Unlike many other areas in health care, the practice of oncology presents unique challenges that make assessing and improving value especially complex. First, patients and professionals feel a well-justified sense of urgency to treat for cure, and if cure is not possible, to extend life and reduce the burden of disease. Second, treatments are often both life sparing and highly toxic (and occasionally life threatening). Third, distinctive payment structures for cancer medicines are intertwined with practice. Fourth, providers often face tremendous pressure to apply the newest technologies to patients who fail to respond to established treatments, even when the evidence supporting those technologies is incomplete or uncertain, and providers may be reluctant to stop toxic treatments and move to palliation, even at the end of life. Finally, the newest and most novel treatments in oncology are among the most costly in medicine.

This report summarizes the results of a workshop that addressed these issues from multiple perspectives, including those of patients and patient advocates, providers, insurers, health care researchers, federal agencies, and industry. Its broad goal was to describe value in oncology in a complete and nuanced way, in order to identify areas of agreement such that a more uniform understanding of value would be available to those faced with decisions regarding developing, evaluating, prescribing, and paying for cancer therapeutics. As the national discussion around health care costs and value continues, a practical working description of value in oncology would benefit many stakeholders and serve as a useful model for other fields of medicine.

The first part of the workshop focused on features of oncology that impact the value proposition. The second part presented potential approaches to improve value in cancer care. During the final session, participants discussed how the concept of value in cancer care is understood now and how it may be understood in the future, exploring any contrasting views and building on areas of agreement.

It is hoped that readers of this will gain insight into the many facets of and challenges to assessing value in cancer care, and perhaps feel the enthusiasm shared by the workshop participants regarding the need to better define value, such that cancer care can improve patients' lives as efficiently and effectively as possible under the reality of the need to control spiraling health care costs.

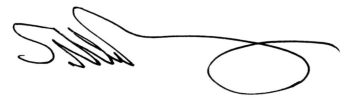

Scott D. Ramsey, M.D., Ph.D.
Chair, Planning Committee on Assessing and Improving Value in Cancer
    Care
Member, National Cancer Policy Forum
Member, Fred Hutchinson Cancer Research Center

1

Introduction

On February 9 and 10, 2009, a public workshop titled Assessing and Improving Value in Cancer Care was presented to the Institute of Medicine's (IOM's) National Cancer Policy Forum[1] (the forum). This workshop was the result of the forum's discussions of value in oncology during meetings held between March 2007 and October 2008. Those discussions, involving forum chair Harold Moses and led by forum members Scott Ramsey, Peter Bach, Betty Ferrell, Roy Herbst, John Niederhuber, Edith Perez, and Ellen Stovall, among others, resulted in the appointment of a planning group led by Scott Ramsey.

During their initial discussions, members of the forum observed that many new treatments in oncology carried increasingly unsustainable eco-

---

[1] The forum was established as a unit of the IOM on May 1, 2005, with support from the following agencies of the U.S. Department of Health and Human Services (HHS): the National Cancer Institute (NCI), the Centers for Disease Control and Prevention (CDC), the Agency for Healthcare Research and Quality (AHRQ), the Food and Drug Administration (FDA), the Centers for Medicare and Medicaid Services (CMS), and the Health Resources and Services Administration (HRSA); as well as from the following private-sector organizations: the American Cancer Society (ACS), the American Society of Clinical Oncology (ASCO), C-Change, and (for the first year only) UnitedHealthcare Group. The forum is a successor to the IOM and National Research Council's (NRC's) National Cancer Policy Board (1997–2005) and was designed to provide its 21 governmental, industry, and academic members a venue for exchanging information and presenting individual views on emerging policy issues in the nation's effort to combat cancer.

nomic costs, and patients, providers, and payors faced the growing challenge of deciding whether or not the benefits of these treatments justified their expense. A clearer understanding of value in cancer care would be integral to support those decisions, and the forum members recognized that value, which is commonly regarded in health care as the benefits of a treatment weighed against its financial cost, deserves particularly careful consideration in oncology. Value in cancer care, the forum members noted, encompasses complex topics including quality end-of-life care, clinical discussions of health care costs, and evidence for treatment effectiveness, among many others. Dr. Ramsey proposed that the forum provide a vehicle for examination of these issues by holding and reporting a workshop on value in cancer care. Shortly after the workshop was proposed, the planning group was expanded to include the nine members of the planning committee on assessing and improving value in cancer care. The planning committee volunteered to work with IOM staff to organize and lead the workshop, which took place in Washington, DC. Throughout the workshop, attendees from a multitude of fields related to cancer care, health economics, ethics, and public policy engaged with the workshop's two dozen speakers to raise questions, offer thoughts, and contribute suggestions.

This workshop summary details the presentations and discussions that took place during this workshop on assessing and improving value in cancer care. The summary is divided into two parts, matching the format of the workshop itself. The first part focuses on the features of oncology that affect the value proposition and the second part presents viable solutions to improve value in cancer care. The final chapter discusses how value in cancer care can be understood, logical next steps, and ways to promote value in oncology. In addition to informing the forum, this published summary is provided to deliver the information and views that emerged from the workshop to a wider public audience for further dialogue or as an opening to additional IOM study in the future.

2

Opening Remarks:
What Is Value in Cancer Care
and Why Is It Important?

This is a unique economic time in America, and health care is intertwined with our broader economic difficulties, said Dr. Scott Ramsey of the Fred Hutchinson Cancer Research Center. Oncology spending is growing at more than 15 percent annually, faster than total health spending and much faster than total United States gross domestic product (GDP). As a result, oncology patients are feeling the pinch, and cost considerations are becoming increasingly intrusive concerns for patients, providers, and payors alike. Much of this spending in oncology is driven by three factors:

- Less expensive treatments are being replaced with more expensive treatments with varying degrees of effectiveness.
- Physicians are being more aggressive in the amount of treatment and treatment combinations given to cancer patients.
- Because patients are living longer, the period of treatment is being prolonged as well.

In oncology, there are certain factors that discourage consideration of evidence concerning safety, effectiveness, and cost-effectiveness. Cancer patients perceive that they are in life-threatening situations, often correctly. This creates urgency that can drive the use of technologies with less evidence for their effectiveness, and patients and physicians in this situation may discount the harms of treatments when they perceive that the only alternative is usual care with a known mortality risk. Some view cost concerns as unimportant, or even inappropriate and offensive, when considering treatments that might improve survival. In addition, the health care delivery system's incentives favor treatment over many other important steps, such as providing patients further information, comfort measures, or end-of-life planning, and these may take second place to costly interventions.

The task set out for this workshop by the planning committee is to address issues related to value in cancer care by identifying agreement in our understanding of value and providing policy tools that can lead to improvements in the value of cancer services provided to patients, said Dr. Ramsey. It is important to discuss terminology used to describe value and the metrics used to measure it, since discussion becomes difficult without a mutual understanding of what is meant by the term *value*. There is no one description of value that everyone agrees on, which is why it is important to understand what constitutes value from the perspectives of many stakeholders—patients, clinicians, payors, industry, and others. We hope that a greater understanding of value from various perspectives will help us jointly weigh the costs of treatments with their risks and benefits.

Many descriptions of value have been proposed previously and may be useful for understanding value in cancer care. Definitions of value in the Merriam-Webster dictionary (Value, 2009) focus largely on a return for a cost in terms of goods or services. They often focus on money, worth, and numerical quantity. This parallels themes at issue for value in oncology—relative worth, fair return, costs, and measures of quality.

Health systems in countries worldwide have described value so that stakeholders in these countries have a common framework for discussion. The European Observatory on Health Systems and Policies (Sorenson et al., 2008) describes value as follows: "Value includes patient preferences, quality, equity, efficiency, and product acceptability among a wide range of stakeholders." Interestingly, cost is not explicitly mentioned here. The United Kingdom's National Institute for Health and Clinical Excellence (NICE) states, "The value of a treatment is based on scientific value judgments, including clinical evaluation and an economic evaluation, and social value judgments, including considerations of efficiency and effectiveness" (Rawlins, 2004). Notice that it focuses on scientific and clinical judgments, and that economics, social judgments, efficiency, and effectiveness are also included. In the United States, Pharmaceutical Research and Manufacturers of America (PhRMA) states that "The value of new and better medicine stems not only from the improved treatment of disease but also from a reduction in other health care costs, increased productivity, and better quality of life" (PhRMA, 2006).

Dr. Ramsey explained that a survey had been distributed to the speakers before the workshop asking them to describe value in cancer care in one sentence. The survey responses were quite varied. Dr. Ramsey presented common concepts, domains, and metrics identified by the informal speaker survey. Concepts and domains included duration and quality of life, health status, cost, equity, compassion, and opportunity. Metrics included quality-adjusted life-years (QALYs), efficiency, effectiveness, necessity, reasonableness, and affordability (Table 2-1). Dr. Ramsey ended his opening comments by emphasizing the variety of conceptions and metrics of value found in this survey of just the workshop's small group of speakers.

TABLE 2-1 Concepts, Domains, Metrics, and Assessments of Value Identified in an Informal Survey of Workshop Speakers

Concepts and Domains
Duration of life
Quality of life
Health Status
Cost
Quality of care
Equity
Compassion
Opportunity

Metrics and Assessments
QALYs
Cost per QALY
Cost for quality
Efficiency
Effectiveness
Necessity
Reasonableness
Affordability

SOURCE: Ramsey presentation, February 9, 2009.

REFERENCES

PhRMA (Pharmaceutical Research and Manufacturers of America). 2006. *Value of medicines: Facts and figures 2006.* Washington, DC: Pharmaceutical Research and Manufacturers of America.

Rawlins, M. 2004. *Scientific and social value judgements.* London, UK: National Institute for Clinical Excellence.

Sorenson, C., M. Drummond, and P. Kanavos. 2008. *Ensuring value for money in health care: The role of health technology assessment in the European Union.* Copenhagen, Denmark: The European Observatory on Health Systems and Policies.

Value. 2009. *Merriam-Webster online dictionary.* http://www.merriam-webster.com/value (accessed April 28, 2009).

PART I:

Challenges to Value in Cancer Care

3

Clinician–Patient Communication and Its Influence on Value

A panel of experts discussed communication in the clinic and at the hospital bedside and its influence on value. Clinician–patient discussions, effective communication with patients about risks and benefits of treatment, and patient expectations during cancer care were discussed to illustrate their effect on value in oncology.

INSIDE THE CLINICIAN–PATIENT DISCUSSION IN CANCER CARE

As a practicing medical oncologist, Dr. Anthony Back of the University of Washington understood how difficult it could be to communicate about cost and value during clinical encounters, he said. His presentation explored the relationship between communication and value by considering transitions to end-of-life care, illustrating communication problems in current practice, presenting views from the patients' perspective, and positing aspects of clinician–patient interaction that confer value. While many in oncology assume that good communication is something that cannot be taught—one is either born with the ability or not—Dr. Back emphasized that communication skills could, in fact, be learned.

Transitions from active anticancer treatment to end-of-life care that assures comfort and prepares the patient and family for death are moments in the trajectory of care that can serve as a useful paradigm for considering clinician–patient interactions and value. Current communication and practice near the end of life can be improved. For instance, a landmark study found that do-not-resuscitate (DNR) orders are written an average of 2 days before death of the patient (SUPPORT Principal Investigators, 1995), and many patients with metastatic cancer are given new active treatment regimens within 2 weeks of death (Harrington and Smith, 2008). While costs increase and treatment too often intensifies at the end of life, Dr. Back explained, what families remember is hearing the message that "There is nothing more to be done" and feeling a sense of abandonment. The clinical reality is one in which doctors are hesitant to be frank with patients and many clinicians behave as though patient well-being will take care of itself if only the right drug is given, with or without discussion. In fact, medical outcomes are highly influenced by communication. Greater communication about transitions to end-of-life care appears to direct subsequent medical care and correlates with lower odds of intensive care unit (ICU) admission, ventilator use, and attempted resuscitation (Wright et al., 2008), as shown in Table 3-1. Without causing increased distress or depression, advance care planning discussions also correlate with greater patient acceptance of terminal illness (Table 3-1), as well as with improved caregiver quality of life, preparation for death, and reduced feelings of regret (Wright et al., 2008).

Despite the importance of these discussions, physicians feel ambivalent toward having them. When asked, doctors feel as though they have no good communication options—they fear taking away hope from patients and families if they do discuss prognosis, but they also know that crucial opportunities to improve care will be missed if these discussions are avoided. Often clinicians have had traumatic experiences in previous discussions of prognosis. This leads to negative emotions toward explicitly discussing prognosis or other difficult topics, and a type of collusion develops between the patient and clinician (The et al., 2000), which Dr. Back phrased "Don't offer, don't dwell."

There is limited data on whether physician discomfort translates into fewer end-of-life discussions, but one study found that medical students maintained greater positive affect[1] if they concealed bad news in simulated encounters with standardized patients compared to those who disclosed

---

[1] Positive affect was measured using the Positive and Negative Affect Scale (Watson et al., 1988). Positive affect is "the conscious subjective aspect of an emotion considered apart from bodily changes" (Affect, 2009).

TABLE 3-1 Outcomes Correlated with an End-of-Life Transition Discussion

Outcomes	Number (percent)			
	End-of-Life Discussion			
	Total Sample (n = 332)	Yes (n = 123)	No (n = 209)	Adjusted OR (95% CI)
Medical care outcomes				
ICU admission	31 (9.3)	5 (4.1)	26 (12.4)	0.35 (0.14–0.90)
Ventilator use	25 (7.5)	2 (1.6)	23 (11.0)	0.26 (0.08–0.83)
Resuscitation attempt	15 (4.5)	1 (0.8)	14 (6.7)	0.16 (0.03–0.80)
Outpatient hospice for over 1 week	173 (52.3)	80 (65.6)	93 (44.5)	1.50 (1.04–2.63)
Mental disorders				
Major depressive disorder	22 (6.7)	10 (8.3)	12 (5.8)	Nonsignificant
Any mental disorder[a]	33 (10.2)	11 (9.2)	22 (10.7)	Nonsignificant
Acceptance of illness as terminal	125 (37.7)	65 (52.9)	60 (28.7)	2.19 (1.40–3.43)
Patient affect score[b]				
Depressed	7.4 (2.9)	7.3 (0.2)	7.4 (0.2)	Nonsignificant
Nervous or worried	6.9 (3.2)	6.5 (0.3)	7.0 (0.3)	Nonsignificant
Sad	7.2 (3.1)	7.3 (0.2)	7.2 (0.2)	Nonsignificant
Terrified	7.2 (3.1)	7.1 (0.3)	7.2 (0.3)	Nonsignificant

[a]Disorders included major depressive disorder, panic disorder, generalized anxiety disorder, and post-traumatic stress disorder.
[b]Assessed using the McGill Psychological Subscale, adjusted least square means.
SOURCES: Back presentation, February 9, 2009; Wright et al., 2008.

the bad news (Panagopoulou et al., 2008). In the study, students were told a piece of bad news about a patient they were asked to interview. When students were told to conceal the bad news and did so, their positive affect decreased before seeing the patient and then rebounded afterward because the encounter had not been as bad as they expected. During encounters in which students disclosed the bad news, their positive affect decreased and remained low (Panagopoulou et al., 2008), as shown in Figure 3-1. Based on these results, Dr. Back posited that it is easier emotionally for clinicians to avoid delivering bad news at the end of life, especially if they are not trained to communicate well in these situations.

For patients, the emotional content of discussions about prognosis or end-of-life transitions can be overwhelming, and they may have difficulty processing prognostic information as a result. Dr. Back recalled a patient who likened receiving bad news to a dump truck unloading its

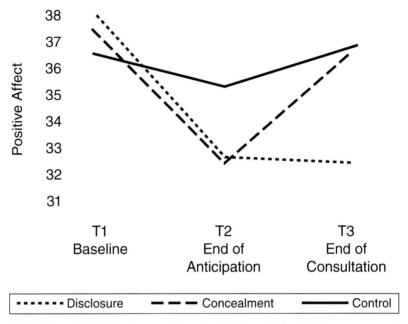

FIGURE 3-1 Medical student positive affect during and after disclosure or conceal-ment of bad news.
SOURCES: Back presentation, February 9, 2009; Panagopoulou et al., 2008.

contents on her front lawn. Oncologists too rarely address this emotional content, however. The largest study of communication with advanced can-cer patients (270 patients, 51 oncologists, and 398 clinic audio recorded visits) found that oncologists made empathic statements to acknowledge emotions patients expressed in only 11 percent of conversations (Pollak et al., 2007). This emotional content is woven into the clinical encounter and addressing it should not be separable from discussions of patients' bio-medical problems.

How long would it take to address patient emotion in a clinical encounter? Not very long, according to a randomized study of women with breast cancer who watched one of two videos of physicians speaking to them, one video with basic empathic language and the other with none. Only 40 seconds of empathic language was required to significantly reduce anxiety among the women (Fogarty et al., 1999). Once the skill of empathic communication is acquired, Dr. Back said, it could be used as part of usual clinical practice without taking much additional time.

Dr. Back then presented data showing that communication skills can be learned. During a four-day workshop on communication tasks, oncology fellows acquired an average of 5.4 skills for delivering bad news and 4.4 skills in transition discussions as assessed by blinded coding of standardized patient encounters (Back et al., 2007). The skills acquired included improvements in fellows' ability to assess patient perceptions, request permission, use the word *cancer* when delivering bad news, make empathic statements after delivering news, elicit patients' reactions, and summarize a follow-up plan (Back et al., 2007), as shown in Figure 3-2. In these standardized encounters, when the patient asked "Isn't there anything more you can do?," fellows initially replied with "You've had a lot of chemotherapy, haven't you?," or similar statements. Dr. Back explained that after the workshop fellows responded more appropriately, saying, for example, "There are more things we can do. Yes, this has been a roller-coaster ride for you, hasn't it?" The fellows had learned to recognize that there were more things that could be done *and* acknowledge the difficult emotions the patient was experiencing. The fellows themselves noticed a difference in their conversations after their training. One said, "I feel less flustered, and my words are less tangled. I can focus on the person across from me and find out what they need from me in that moment, and that seems like progress."

Dr. Back shared insights into what patients want during clinical discussions. Based on results from a series of interviews, it was clear that patients wanted empathy and guidance from their physicians, and they did not want to be abandoned. One patient said that "The doctor has to allow [the patient] to let his emotions run a little bit." Others said "I want to hear all the options," and another was concerned that "There's no leadership or guidance from the doctor." Patients also worried that they would be abandoned by their doctor in the end. During another series of interviews, some patients said, "It's important that doctors still have that contact with patients, even though there isn't anything the doctor can do to make the patient better," or "I need to be able to depend on my doctor. If I call you next week, Doctor, will you see me right away, even if I'm not getting more chemotherapy?"

Closer to death, patients discussed the importance of closure with their doctor (Back et al., 2009). One spouse whose husband died of cancer said, "I realize the doctor is busy, but he knew [the patient] and I. We were together through the whole thing. It would have been nice to hear from him." Their oncologist had referred the patient to hospice, and the family never heard from him again. When this oncologist thought about contacting the fam-

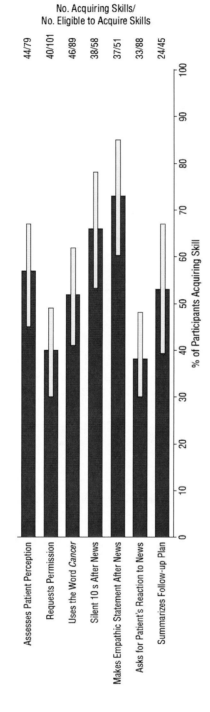

FIGURE 3-2 Fellows' skill acquisition in delivering bad news after a communication workshop.
NOTE: Dark bars indicate the percentage of participants acquiring a skill. Light bars indicate 95% confidence intervals.
SOURCES: Back presentation, February 9, 2009; Back et al., 2007.

ily, he reported, "I felt guilty because I hadn't called her earlier, and I didn't know if it was appropriate. Maybe it would just stir up emotional stuff." The doctor's interpretation minimized the value of what he had to offer the family in that moment, when in fact what he had to offer—communication, nonabandonment, and a sense of closure at the end of life—was exactly what the patient and his bereaved spouse considered highly valuable.

What gives clinician–patient interactions value? Dr. Back explained that the way oncologists communicate creates a framework for defining what is valuable in cancer care. Some aspects of value are immediately obvious, such as access to biomedical therapies and construction of patient hope. However, other aspects of value are only discovered by oncologists through experience and are dependent upon effective communication focused on defining quality of life, handling information, and nonabandonment. Oncologists are not born with the requisite communication skills—communication is clinical work that has to be learned.

What is still missing from clinician–patient communication? Cost discussions, Dr. Back said, which may be because physicians do not know how to talk about financial costs without assuming the role of gatekeepers. Oncologists will have to learn new ways to communicate to bring societal cost issues into clinical discussions.

Invited Response

As a social worker, Ms. Diane Blum of CancerCare said understanding the impact of illness on the patients' families, work, finances, and insurance is integral to practice. Social workers do, in fact, talk about money with patients. Patient values—not just monetary values—are central in all of those discussions.

Good communication is the cornerstone of quality care. As part of quality care, the Institute of Medicine (IOM) report *Cancer Care for the Whole Patient: Meeting Psychosocial Health Needs* (IOM, 2008) recommends a regular assessment of domains of concern to patients, including the emotional capacity of the patient and family, as well as their educational, financial, legal, and work needs. The report lays out the evidence base supporting communication to meet the wider needs of the patient, including the psychosocial needs that very clearly include cost issues. Ms. Blum said that her organization, CancerCare, receives roughly 1,500 calls per week from people asking for help. Fifteen percent of them have a communication need, and 55 percent have a financial need. Sometimes the amount of clinical information can be overwhelming, and discussions of priorities become difficult. For people facing life-threatening illness, communication about the emotional impact of cancer is essential.

For Ms. Blum, a quote from Alice Hoffman captured the emotional impact of cancer well. Written about the moment she learned of her diagnosis, her quote reads:

> I was certain my doctor was phoning me to tell me that the biopsy had come back negative. I was absolutely sure of it. But then she said, "Alice, I'm sorry." I could hear the concern in her voice, and I understood that some things are true, no matter how and when you're told. In a single moment, the world as I knew it dropped away from me, leaving me on a far and distant planet, one where there was no gravity and no oxygen and nothing made sense anymore. (Hoffman, 2000)

This is a powerful reminder of the importance of our words and how much they mean, Ms. Blum said, and the words our culture uses to discuss cancer also deserve attention. Thirty years ago, Susan Sontag wrote about illness as a metaphor (Sontag, 1978), and today the words used to describe illnesses such as cancer carry no less significance. Ms. Blum recalled a magazine article entitled "Patrick Swayze Is Winning His Battle Against Cancer" in which the actor said of his pancreatic cancer, "I'm a miracle, dude" and "I'm going to beat this." Ms. Blum commended Ruth Bader Ginsburg's candor when announcing that she had pancreatic cancer. She had used similar language to describe her "fight" with cancer. Swayze and Ginsburg are emblematic of a culture in which cancer patients are told to fight and struggle and battle, and anything less is seen as weakness. This is difficult to reconcile with discussions of cost, which patients and clinicians must have. How can one worry about costs when the outcome is uncertain? Patients are told to fight for any chance of cure, and anything less than the fullest effort, financial or otherwise, is undignified. Helping patients understand value in their care and putting it in some perspective to aid their decisions is a big task, Ms. Blum said, but she had hope for strategies to make progress.

Invited Response

Language matters. Ms. Mary McCabe of Memorial Sloan-Kettering Cancer Center said she would like to do away with much of the language she hears such as "Do you want me to do everything?" or "There's nothing more we can do." She expressed concern that clinicians, in trying to maintain hope, sometimes inadvertently offer false choices, because they offer medical interventions of little clinical value and leave the decision up to the patient and family without professional guidance regarding what treatments do or do not have potential for benefit.

In her many years as an oncology nurse and an ethics consultant, Ms. McCabe often noticed that patients and their families would talk about their concerns with nurses outside of the exam room, outside of the clinic, or in the hospital hall after the physicians had left. The questions often involved how to maximize quality of life in the time remaining and sometimes included the issue of cost of treatment and care. These are the conversations that need to be brought back into the room before the physician leaves. Too often, clinical teams, patients, and families encounter conflicts at the end of life because the conversations that should have taken place never did, or they become subsumed within other very urgent discussions, such as the discussion to obtain a do-not-resuscitate order. This is not the time for discussions about costs and quality of life.

In closing, Ms. McCabe emphasized that value is decided at the bedside. It is where the rubber hits the road. In the context of limited resources, rather than thinking about bedside decisions regarding cost as "rationing," it is essential to frame them in the positive, toward value.

THERAPY FOR ADVANCED-STAGE CANCER: WHAT DO PATIENTS WANT AND EXPECT?

People with cancer want to live, Mr. Robert Erwin of the Marti Nelson Cancer Foundation said. Everyone who is first diagnosed with advanced cancer—at the first recurrence or sign that their therapy will not work—still has hope for meaningful life extension. But when is this hope realistic and when is hope false? One cannot really judge whether hope is realistic or false except in retrospect. Nevertheless, false hope is likely driven by a constant drumbeat of optimism for cure that is frequently misguided and overstated. Another driver is incomplete patient information. Possible sources of information are many, and there is often too little time for patients to review and understand them all, whether during a clinical encounter or at other times. Outright fraud masquerading as effective treatment can also drive false hope, taking advantage of the sense that cures for advanced cancer must exist and can be found if one just looks hard enough. There is value in hope—realistic hope in particular.

The value of hope implies value in the *opportunity* for life extension, whether a positive outcome is realized or not. The cost of therapy, price of the drug, and the hospital fees are not valuable just because they work for some people. They also provide an opportunity for everyone who elects to try that therapy, drug, or hospital care. This is what drives many patients and providers to continue treatment even after the first or the second or the third has failed. While the results of randomized controlled trials (RCTs) are held out as the gold standard of clinical evidence, the selected populations they study and their results do not necessarily predict what will happen when the same treatments are adopted in the real world. The RCTs also present their data in terms of means or medians, which are statistical abstractions from a population. Therefore they cannot perfectly predict the outcome for any individual patient. As a result, patients may not be satisfied to simply take the results of the RCTs as gospel. This view is supported by the surprising increased survival results of the large-scale, observational BRiTE study recently published by Grothey and colleagues (Grothey et al., 2008).

There is also value in eliminating options early on, getting rid of fantasies, and moving past unrealistic treatment possibilities. Ultimately, there is value for both the patient and for the family in believing that every reasonable option has been tried.

When treatments are not effective, continuation of treatment is often described in terms of a war or a battle with cancer. Oncologists talk about their "arsenal" to treat patients, and success is described as a "victory" or "fighting on." When treatments are not effective, some say that a patient "failed" a treatment. Death is equated with defeat, but this should not be. After all, death is a natural consequence of life, and everyone is terminal. Does this mean that all of us and all of our physicians will fail when we die? No. Treatments fail, not patients or their physicians. Therefore, at certain stages of the cancer care process when further active anticancer treatment is no longer useful, perhaps other terms are more appropriate, such as "peace," "preparation for death," and "acceptance."

Discussions of family relationships and the things that people want to do or say before death are also important, but sometimes people need permission to pursue them, Mr. Erwin said. They need encouragement to have those discussions and leave their family slightly more happily than if they were compelled to fight to the bitter end in a coma or the ICU rather than at home or in hospice.

Patients want to live—to return to health and a normal life. Sometimes they get it, sometimes they do not, and what they want may change to just a desire for a few more years or months. Patients always want hope, if not for more life then at least for a good quality of life in the time remaining. Patients certainly want truth from the very beginning, even if they do not understand what is being said; they will understand the truth eventually anyway. Patients want dignity, the absence of pain, and what some call "a good death." As a society, we need to consider how we can protect vulnerable people from exploitation and increase the value we place on engaging with death as a natural and unavoidable consequence of life. If we can both empower people to be aggressive when it is appropriate but also empower them to accept what is naturally going to happen, we will have achieved better value in cancer care.

DISCUSSION

Dr. Thomas Smith of the Massey Cancer Center mentioned previous work indicating that patients are more comfortable discussing advance directives with admitting hospitalists than in more established relationships with their oncologists. He asked whether it could be that the closer one is with the clinician, the more uncomfortable the advance directive discussion becomes. Are information brokers needed for these conversations outside of the clinician–patient relationship? Dr. Back wondered if the findings reflected ways in which oncologists and patients construct their relationships. He saw these relationship dynamics as potentially changeable and was not sure if a third party with a different level of training would solve the problem or simply complicate the situation.

Dr. Betty Ferrell of City of Hope commented on policy remedies to improve value in cancer care, saying that Americans with advanced lung, pancreatic, ovarian, and other cancers are effectively denied access to hospice care because of the current reimbursement system, and many more hospitals could improve the quality of the care they deliver if reimbursement was realigned to cover pain management and psychosocial and palliative care services necessary for high-quality care. Ms. Ellen Stovall agreed, saying that she often feels as though reimbursement reforms are accomplished piecemeal by retrofitting an already very broken system. Reimbursement should be provided to match and follow the services that have been defined as high quality in the cancer care community. Right now that alignment does not exist.

Dr. Lee Newcomer of UnitedHealthcare pointed out that patients routinely budget to make many decisions—hamburger versus steak, new car versus used car, and other things they can or cannot afford. Patients already understand and discuss costs in these ways. So why is it more difficult for patients to discuss medical costs? Dr. Back thought these discussions were possible, but the framework for considering large-scale societal costs in the context of a clinical encounter did not yet exist. In the United States, doctors too often discuss costs as gatekeepers—"You can't have this"—and this shapes how patients view the cost discussion. What needs to be developed is an appreciation of the societal value and shared benefit that we can protect by discussing cost in health care. This is the challenge.

REFERENCES

Affect. 2009. *Merriam-Webster online dictionary.* http://www.merriam-webster.com/dictionary/affect (accessed August 14, 2009).

Back, A. L., R. M. Arnold, W. F. Baile, K. A. Fryer-Edwards, S. C. Alexander, G. E. Barley, T. A. Gooley, and J. A. Tulsky. 2007. Efficacy of communication skills training for giving bad news and discussing transitions to palliative care. *Archives of Internal Medicine* 167(5):453–460.

Back, A. L., J. P. Young, E. McCown, R. Engelberg, E. K. Vig, L. F. Reinke, M. D. Wenrich, B. B. McGrath, and R. J. Curtis. 2009. Abandonment at the end of life from patient, caregiver, nurse, and physician perspectives: Loss of continuity and lack of closure. *Archives of Internal Medicine* 169(5):474–479.

Fogarty, L. A., B. A. Curbow, J. R. Wingard, K. McDonnell, and M. R. Somerfield. 1999. Can 40 seconds of compassion reduce patient anxiety? *Journal of Clinical Oncology* 17(1):371–379.

Grothey, A., M. M. Sugrue, D. M. Purdie, D. Sargent, E. Hedrick, and M. Kozloff. 2008. Bevacizumab beyond first progression is associated with prolonged overall survival in metastatic colorectal cancer: Results from a large observational cohort study (BRiTE). *Journal of Clinical Oncology* 26(33):5326–5334.

Harrington, S. E., and T. J. Smith. 2008. The role of chemotherapy at the end of life: "When is enough, enough?" *Journal of the American Medical Association* 299(22):2667–2678.

Hoffman, A. 2000. Sustained by fiction while facing life's facts. *The New York Times*, August 14, 2000.

IOM (Institute of Medicine). 2008. *Cancer care for the whole patient: Meeting psychosocial health needs.* Washington, DC: The National Academies Press.

Panagopoulou, E., G. Mintziori, A. Montgomery, and D. Kapoukranidou. 2008. Concealment of information in clinical practice: Is lying less stressful than telling the truth? *Journal of Clinical Oncology* 26(7):1175–1177.

Pollak, K. I., R. M. Arnold, A. S. Jeffreys, S. C. Alexander, M. K. Olsen, A. P. Abernathy, C. S. Skinner, K. L. Rodriguez, and J. A. Tulsky. 2007. Oncologist communication about emotion during visits with patients with advanced cancer. *Journal of Clinical Oncology* 25(36):5748–5752.

Sontag, S. 1978. *Illness as metaphor.* New York: Farrar, Strauss, Giroux.

SUPPORT Principal Investigators. 1995. A controlled trial to improve care for seriously ill hospitalized patients. The Study to Understand Prognoses and Preferences for Outcomes and Risks of Treatments (SUPPORT). *Journal of the American Medical Association* 274(20):1591–1598.

The, A.-M., T. Hak, G. Koeter, and G. van der Wal. 2000. Collusion in doctor-patient communication about imminent death: An ethnographic study. *BMJ* 321(7273):1376–1381.

Watson, D., L. A. Clark, and A. Tellegen. 1988. Development and validation of brief measures of positive and negative affect: The PANAS scales. *Journal of Personality and Social Psychology* 54(6):1063–1070.

Wright, A. A., B. Zhang, A. Ray, J. W. Mack, E. Trice, T. Balboni, S. L. Mitchell, V. A. Jackson, S. D. Block, P. K. Maciejewski, and H. G. Prigerson. 2008. Associations between end-of-life discussions, patient mental health, medical care near death, and caregiver bereavement adjustment. *Journal of the American Medical Association* 300(14):1665–1673.

4

Generating Evidence About Effectiveness and Value

Dr. Steven Cohen of the Agency for Healthcare Research and Quality (AHRQ) introduced a second panel of experts to discuss evidence for effectiveness and value.

THE FDA AND EVIDENCE FOR REGULATORY APPROVAL IN CANCER

The Food and Drug Administration (FDA) operates at the introduction of cancer care drugs and biological therapeutics into the market, Dr. Janet Woodcock of the FDA's Center for Drug Evaluation and Research said. What role does the FDA review process play for value in cancer care?

Before the FDA efficacy standard was put into place in the 1960s, the requirement that a drug show benefit to patients before reaching the market was very controversial. Since that time, the FDA has required that treatments reaching the market demonstrate evidence of effectiveness—defined as benefit to the patient, not to doctors or to society at large. This requirement that drugs and biologics in the market demonstrate clinical benefit and safety, has been one of the most significant drivers of treatment evidence in medicine.

To determine clinical benefit, the FDA has considered the endpoints of survival extension, improvement in function, and quality of life as a result of a drug, but the FDA has never considered cost-effectiveness. If a drug provides longer life, better function, or better quality of life, the FDA would approve it regardless of its cost.

In oncology presently, survival and improvement in patient-reported symptoms are considered unequivocally while weighing a drug's clinical benefits. Other measures may be included as well, such as objective response rate and time to progression. While the FDA is very supportive of using health-related quality of life as an endpoint, generating the evidence has proved difficult, and few drugs have reached the market based only on this measure. Blinding is difficult in trials to determine health-related quality of life; very careful serial assessments are essential, and the clinical significance to patients of changes in quality of life may be unclear or of little utility compared to careful recording of toxicity data. In combination with objective antitumor effects, the quality-of-life outcomes are more credible. Nevertheless, it is hoped that advances will be made in methods for generating accurate health-related quality-of-life data, said Dr. Woodcock.

Many drugs reaching the market in recent decades have been approved after regulations were implemented allowing approval based on surrogate endpoints (accelerated approval). Put in place during the HIV epidemic, these regulations were set up for serious and life-threatening diseases in which a drug appears to provide benefit over existing therapies based on a surrogate endpoint thought to reasonably predict clinical benefit. Accelerated approval has been used extensively in cancer drug approvals in recent years. Accelerated approval is subject to legal requirements that the applicant complete longer-term postmarketing studies to verify and describe the clinical benefit of their drug. These postmarketing studies should usually be underway at the time of approval. Therefore the value of therapies approved this way is not fully clear at the time of launch and may remain unclear until confirmatory studies are complete.

Recently, time to tumor progression, or progression-free survival, has been suggested as a measure of clinical benefit. Often, time to progression involves measuring radiographic or other evidence of progression. Clearly, if tumor progression occurs, it will eventually lead to negative outcomes, but this must also be weighed against the harm a treatment may cause. This leads to more uncertainty than measuring objective survival (Table 4-1). Ultimately, the importance of time to progression depends on the size of the benefit. If the benefit is large and unequivocal, then our uncertainty is low. If the difference is only apparent statistically with equivocal impact on patient well-being, then the benefit of the drug remains quite uncertain, and the evidence is much less persuasive for approval.

TABLE 4-1 Comparison of Two Measures of Benefit in FDA Approval: Overall Survival and Time to Tumor Progression

Overall Survival	Time to Tumor Progression
Perfectly accurate event	Less accurate event
Perfectly accurate time	Less accurate time
Assessed daily or more frequently	Assessed every 2–6 months
Unquestioned importance	Uncertain importance
Measure of safety and efficacy	Measure of efficacy only
Longer time to reach endpoint	Shorter time to reach endpoint
May be obscured by secondary interventions	Not obscured by secondary interventions

SOURCE: Woodcock presentation, February 9, 2009.

Response rate as a surrogate measure provides even less certainty of clinical benefit. When considering approval based on response rate, important questions remain. For instance, what was the number of complete responses compared to partial responses? What was the duration of response and anatomical location? Were they associated with symptom improvement or the extent of metastatic disease? These details matter.

Dr. Woodcock reiterated that the FDA has felt pressure to adopt many of these surrogate measures and to consider them measures of full clinical benefit. However, part of achieving value is reducing the uncertainty around treatments that reach the market—people want to know exactly what these drugs can do.

The Shape of Cancer Therapeutics to Come

Fewer than 5 percent of cancer therapeutics entering phase I trials reach the market, the worst track record of any therapeutic area. While pharmaceutical discovery and candidate selection in cancer is driven by recent scientific discoveries, much more of clinical oncology treatment development is empirical—trial and error—compared to other disease therapeutics areas. This approach limits understanding of cancer drug benefits, since there are no means of assessing drugs' pharmacodynamic effect.

The good news, said Dr. Woodcock, is that cancer is probably the most active area in drug development, with many new cancer drugs coming to market. Between July 2005 and December 2007, the FDA approved 53 new indications in oncology, with 18 new molecular entity approvals and 35 supplemental applications (new drug applications or biologic license applications). In recent years, the FDA has only approved 18 new molecular entities annually overall, which means that oncology has been taking the lion's share. FDA has also seen a huge increase in investigational agents studied in cancer, from 925 investigational new drug applications in 2003 to 1,440 in 2008. The question remains: what is their value?

Among the 53 new indications approved by the FDA in cancer therapeutics between July 2005 and December 2007, 38 clearly showed clinical benefit and proceeded through the approval process using regular approval indications, while 10 used accelerated approval, and 5 previous accelerated approvals were converted to regular approvals upon completion of confirmatory trials with a new indication. With respect to the measures used to support these approvals, 10 indications showed benefits in overall survival, 5 indications were approved based on evidence of disease-free survival, 12 indications were approved based on evidence of time-to-progression or progression-free survival, 17 indications were approved based on response rates, and other, novel endpoints, such as reduction in hepatic iron and depletion of asparagines, were used in the remainder of cases.

While novel therapies that provide benefits are desired by everyone, concerns exist over health care expenditures and whether or not each novel therapy has needed value, Dr. Woodcock said. But most oncology drugs do not benefit exposed patients uniformly, and many nonresponders only experience the drug toxicities, making the benefit-to-risk ratio quite unfavorable in some cases. Safety problems also decrease value when patient injury or inconvenience reduce quality and raise costs to the health care system. Currently, there is little ability to predict who is going to respond to treatment and who will be harmed.

One solution, said Dr. Woodcock, may be the development of predictive biomarkers to improve treatment effectiveness, efficacy, or the size of the treatment effect. Genomic markers for tumor susceptibility, imaging technologies for superior assessment of tumor response, proteomic markers for tumor subcategorization, and the use of circulating tumor cells are all promising avenues for predictive biomarker development. There is reason for some skepticism about the value of these technologies because of their added cost, but if they provide the ability to spare many patients from therapy that will not benefit them, the result will be a tremendous savings. Tailoring treatment in this way is also simply the right thing to do for patients.

Predictive biomarkers for safety are already being implemented in oncology. Drug-metabolizing enzyme variants and drug-transporter variants are used to predict the total exposure of the patient or their cellular exposure to an agent. Currently, the maximum tolerated dose in groups of patients in phase I trials are examined, but the underlying mechanistic reasons why some groups within the population may not tolerate the therapy are not identified. This may lead to underdosing of many patients because a smaller subset with a distinct variant biomarker is very sensitive to the therapy, and standard dosages are set to those outliers. If these variants can be used to avoid serious side effects of treatments in some patients, their use can improve value.

Many challenges for oncology will accompany the large number of candidate drugs arriving soon. The FDA does not have a cost-effectiveness standard for putting these drugs on the market, and the community will have to sort out the ones that are truly valuable.

In conclusion, Dr. Woodcock reiterated that drug development leading to FDA approval is an important step in evidence development for cancer drugs. For many cancer drugs, it is the only rigorous evidence development process in place. FDA approval is predicated on showing that a treatment's effectiveness outweighs its harm, harm which may be significant in cancer therapy. Finally, many new methods of targeting therapy could increase value significantly by increasing the size of treatment effects and decreasing the amount of harm.

WHAT CONSTITUTES REASONABLE EVIDENCE OF EFFICACY AND EFFECTIVENESS IN CANCER CARE?

In the treatment of life-threatening diseases, there is a pressure to adopt new treatments based on less evidence, and treatment risks may be discounted when the alternative is death. This can make meeting the standard of "reasonable" and "logical" treatment more difficult in cancer care.

Dr. Daniel Sargent of the Mayo Clinic defined a few key terms to begin to address the question he set out to answer through his presentation, "What constitutes reasonable evidence of efficacy and effectiveness in cancer care?" *Evidence* is "that which tends to prove or disprove something, grounds for belief or proof" (Evidence, 2009). Regarding criteria for evidence, Dr. Sargent emphasized the difficulty in achieving absolute certainty in cancer research, saying that a P-value less than 0.05 still allows a 1 in 20 chance that a finding is a false positive. In addition, clinical cancer research does not occur in a laboratory. The experiments that are possible in clinical trials may not provide perfect evidence to answer all of the important questions. Finally, evidence is often unavailable, inconclusive, or contradictory.

Efficacy is defined as "the capacity for producing a desired result or effect" (Efficacy, 2009). What is the desired result? Is it a full clinical benefit endpoint or a surrogate? Can it be measured precisely and reliably? Is the result that is observed in a particular trial transferable to other settings, such as those in the community? These are all challenges for establishing efficacy, Dr. Sargent said.

Currently, the FDA determines whether evidence for cancer treatment efficacy is reasonable on scientific grounds with appropriate input from patients and often guided by the Oncologic Drug Advisory Committee. Once the FDA gives its blessing, oncologists in the community decide whether evidence for a treatment is actually sufficient to change practice based on guidelines, relevant literature, marketing, and other resources that may represent a different standard than that required for drug approval. Dr. Sargent asked, is the current practice for evaluating efficacy reasonable? Yes, he said, because there is input from many parties, it is gathered in an organized manner, and there are clear, well-accepted standards by which therapies must demonstrate efficacy.

What about effectiveness? *Effectiveness* is defined as "how well a treatment works in practice," as opposed to efficacy, which measures how well a treatment works in a controlled trial. In most cases, oncology trials do not evaluate how well therapies actually work in the community, and clear standards to judge effectiveness are lacking. While there is input from many parties, collection and reporting of treatment effectiveness data are disorganized, and effectiveness is often unclear because therapies are used in situations beyond those examined in clinical trials.

Randomized controlled trials (RCTs) are considered the gold standard of evidence because randomization, intended to balance known and unknown confounding factors between the study groups, allows for causal inference. However, not everything can be randomized, and there are other forms of analysis, such as propensity scores or other statistical modeling adjustments for differences in the treatments received that may facilitate causal inference in nonrandomized settings. For these approaches we can measure as many covariates as we like, but unfortunately we often do not understand many of the covariates that ultimately determine why patients do well or do not, Dr. Sargeant said. Whenever possible, randomized data should be sought.

Dr. Sargent then listed the critical components of a randomized trial, which include:

- Designation of prespecified hypotheses with primary and secondary endpoints;
- Prespecified data cutoffs for any continuous measurement to define what constitutes a positive or negative finding;
- A defined sample set with eligibility criteria that are as inclusive as possible;
- Power calculations to show that there is a reasonable probability of definitively answering the research questions at issue before the experiment is begun;
- Unbiased ascertainment of endpoints, including blinding whenever possible and ethical, protocol-specified criteria, and independent review of endpoints; and
- Complete information through a standard follow-up schedule and with few patients lost to follow-up.

After new therapies are validated as being efficacious in RCTs using these principles, the same treatments are then refined and further studied by the community where the controlled study environment is lost. Doses and schedules are changed. Combinations are made with other agents, or the interventions are used in an off-label manner for other indications. These refinements are rarely studied rigorously, though comparative effectiveness research, meta-analyses, or large-scale observational studies may provide them some level of validation. Because tools for studying treatments in the community are limited in these ways, Dr. Sargent said, this largely prohibits the generation of level I evidence of treatment effectiveness (Table 4-2). How can this gap be bridged?

Two solutions are certainly not new but continue to be underused: (1) cluster randomization and (2) large simple (or pragmatic) trials. When it is impossible to randomize individual patients, one can randomize groups by physician, institution, or geographic area. This is cluster randomization. Large, simple trials use streamlined trial designs with no extra investigations and minimal extra workload. One such trial, the QUASAR (QUick And Simple And Reliable) trial (2007), included roughly 7,000 patients and compared approved regimens of 5-fluorouracil and leucovorin for the treatment of stage II and stage III colon cancer. The eligibility criteria included a diagnosis of colon cancer, patient consent, and no obvious contraindica-

TABLE 4-2 Levels of Evidence and Sources of Evidence to Generate Them

Level of Evidence	Evidence Source
Level I	Evidence from at least one properly randomized, controlled trial
Level II-1	Evidence from well-designed controlled trials without randomization
Level II-2	Evidence from well-designed cohort or case-control analytic studies
Level II-3	Evidence from multiple time series with or without the intervention
Level III	Opinions of authorities, clinical experience; descriptive studies and case reports; reports of expert committees

SOURCES: Sargent presentation, February 9, 2009; Harris et al., 2001.

tions. During the trial, investigators notified the trial office of only serious, unexpected adverse events. Follow-up was yearly to collect data on serious toxicity, recurrence, and death. The study showed benefit of chemotherapy over observation in patients with stage II colon cancer. Economic analyses, compliance, toxicity, and quality-of-life measures were assessed only in a substudy of 600 patients (QUASAR Collaborative Group, 2007). To put large, simple trials into practice requires the use of multicenter trials, minimal patient eligibility criteria, intention-to-treat analyses, and minimization of disincentives to data accrual.

Dr. Sargent turned to a discussion of how evidence can be evaluated based on a hierarchy of endpoint strength. When evaluating evidence for treatments, true clinical efficacy measures, such as overall survival, are always the gold standard. In some cases a validated surrogate endpoint[1] showing effectiveness can predict the true clinical benefit endpoint measure, but this represents a weaker source of evidence than true clinical efficacy measures. The FDA's accelerated approval process uses surrogate endpoints

---

[1] "Validated" surrogate endpoints are determined as follows: the effect of a given intervention on a validated surrogate endpoint reliably predicts the effect of that intervention on the final clinical endpoint of interest. This validation can be accomplished through statistical methods, meta-analyses of RCTs, and the use of clinical information based on the biological disease pathway or the intervention's mechanism of action. For instance, recommendations from the ACCENT group established a new surrogate endpoint in the adjuvant setting for colon cancer through data from 18 previous randomized trials (Sargent et al., 2007). Similar analyses are now underway for surrogates in other diseases, including advanced colon cancer and advanced breast cancer.

that are less validated or "reasonably likely" to predict clinical benefit. The lowest-strength evidence is provided by correlate endpoints that solely measure biological activity of the intervention.

In the future, biomarkers will likely define patient populations based on both risk and potential benefit, and biomarkers will likely allow early assessment of treatment efficacy, both as trial endpoints and as patient-management tools. This has clear value implications, but very few potential biomarkers have been developed to the point of allowing them to be reliably used in clinical practice. Predictive biomarker validation will require randomized clinical trials, either through targeted selection trials (where only patients who express a given biomarker are enrolled) or through unselective enrollment trials with prospectively specified biomarker analysis. While analyses of data from previously conducted trials may also be used to validate biomarkers, the quality of the data may be questionable without standardized protocols and analyses.

As a medical community, Dr. Sargent concluded, we do a reasonable job in determining efficacy, though it is costly, data collection is burdensome, and we need further work to develop reliable early endpoints. However, we rarely collect data to reliably determine effectiveness. Carefully generated experiments are critical to generate this evidence, and large, simple trials and cluster randomization can provide some of this data to bridge the gap between efficacy and effectiveness.

DISCUSSION

Dr. Sean Tunis of the Center for Medical Technology Policy commented on trials to better understand effectiveness, saying that there needs to be a model for simpler trial designs that are more pragmatic and effectiveness oriented. Frequently companies are hesitant to pursue these types of studies for two reasons: (1) they worry that the FDA will impede the studied drug over safety or toxicity issues that may emerge, and (2) they are concerned that there are many more restrictions on marketing of treatments whose effects are determined through studies that are not performed under a traditional regulatory paradigm. How can companies move past such concerns?

Dr. Woodcock responded by saying that it is "almost unheard of" that a cancer drug is delayed because of toxicities in less-controlled trial settings, and some cancer drugs have reached the market based on information gained through access trials with levels of control similar to the large, simple trials. Regarding the legal restrictions on marketing, there is talk in Congress about removing them. The question is this: what evidentiary standards are required for secondary indications, not drug approval? Dr. Woodcock felt that the FDA would be hard-pressed to accept observational studies. They simply do not provide the level of evidence needed to change the medication label. However, clearly more discussion is required about the amount of data needed and ways to increase the size of large, simple trials to support follow-on indications for a cancer drug. Dr. Cohen said that this calls for a sustained commitment to investment in the methodological infrastructure for such trials.

Dr. Martin Murphy of the CEO Roundtable on Cancer asked the panelists about opportunities to retrospectively mine previous clinical trial data to look for signals that might be useful to identify new therapeutics. Dr. Woodcock agreed that the idea was promising and said this would be important for many diseases, especially cancer.

REFERENCES

Efficacy. 2009. *Dictionary.com Unabridged. Random House, Inc.* http://dictionary.reference. com/browse/efficacy (accessed February 9, 2009).

Evidence. 2009. *Dictionary.com Unabridged. Random House, Inc.* http://dictionary.reference. com/browse/evidence (accessed February 9, 2009).

Harris, R. P., M. Helfand, S. H. Woolf, K. N. Lohr, C. D. Mulrow, S. M. Teutsch, D. Atkins, and Methods Work Group of the Third U.S. Preventive Services Task Force. 2001. Current methods of the U.S. Preventive Services Task Force: A review of the process. *American Journal of Preventive Medicine* 20(3 Suppl):21–35.

QUASAR Collaborative Group, R. Gray, J. Barnwell, C. McConkey, R. K. Hills, N. S. Williams, and P. J. Kerr. 2007. Adjuvant chemotherapy versus observation in patients with colorectal cancer: A randomised study. *Lancet* 370(9604):2020–2029.

Sargent, D., S. Patiyil, G. Yothers, D. G. Haller, R. Gray, J. Benedetti, M. Buyse, R. Labianca, J. F. Seitz, C. J. O'Callaghan, G. Francini, A. Grothey, M. O'Connell, P. J. Catalano, D. Kerr, E. Green, H. S. Wieand, R. M. Goldberg, and A. de Gramont. 2007. End points for colon cancer adjuvant trials: Observations and recommendations based on individual patient data from 20,898 patients enrolled onto 18 randomized trials from the ACCENT group. *Journal of Clinical Oncology* 25(29):4569–4574.

5

Value and the Oncology Market

Dr. Jeffrey Lerner of the ECRI Institute (formerly the Emergency Care Research Institute) introduced a panel of expert speakers on pricing for oncology therapies and the economic market in cancer care. The three speakers would discuss the price of medical care, a topic too few discussed in the past, Dr. Lerner said. Instead of thinking about cost and price as secondary issues, perhaps it was time to take them into account through serious science and research, and to count them as part of the value equation.

DRUG PRICING AND VALUE IN ONCOLOGY COMPARED TO OTHER AREAS IN MEDICINE

Dr. Patricia Danzon of the University of Pennsylvania's Wharton School began by describing how she and other economists use the term *value*. To economists, maximizing value from the resources used on all goods and services in the economy, termed economic efficiency, requires that the value gained per dollar spent is equalized across all the ways in which those resources are used. If a bigger "bang for the buck" can be obtained from one use compared to another, there is benefit to be gained by simply transferring resources to the more efficient use, whether in health care versus other economic sectors, oncology versus other medical fields, or certain drugs versus other services within oncology. To achieve this, economists normally rely on incentives to drive efficient resource allocation, but in health care we have to rely on other drivers of value, Dr. Danzon said.

In most markets, the price system, or what Adam Smith called "the invisible hand," drives efficient allocation of resources. The basic idea is simple: consumers make choices—votes with their dollars for the prices they are willing to pay. Consumer "willingness to pay" conveys to manufacturers the value they place on different resources, and this creates an incentive for manufacturers to align their prices with how much consumers are willing to pay. Market prices assure efficient resource allocation only if consumers are well informed, consumers face the full social costs of services (there are no externalities), and the population distribution of consumer income is appropriate or balanced. In this type of well-functioning price system there would be no need to study cost-effectiveness.

With health insurance in place, however, prices are not constrained by consumer willingness to pay. Health insurance exists for a very good reason: to protect us from financial risk that might otherwise be economically catastrophic. In this sense, it is extremely valuable. But insurance undermines patient price sensitivity and leads to "moral hazard" that drives higher volumes and prices of services. Systems of consumer co-payment and cost sharing can mitigate moral hazard, but for many services the cost shares are relatively low as a percent of total cost, and stop-loss measures are in place as an upper limit on a patient's cost share. Therefore, these mechanisms are limited in their ability to sensitize patients to costs.

Less widely studied than moral hazard is the effect of insurance on producer pricing. On the consumer demand curve for medical care with no insurance in place, consumers use fewer services because they pay higher prices. In that situation, a manufacturer would charge a price (P_1; see Figure 5-1) based on the intersection of the marginal revenue and marginal cost curves. When consumers are given insurance coverage with a 50 percent coinsurance rate, the manufacturer's price can be twice as high, as far as the consumer is concerned, because the consumer is only paying half the total price. With this 50 percent coinsurance or co-pay, the manufacturer's price would increase (P_2), and a higher quantity (Q_2 compared to Q_1) can be sold because consumers pay less of the price. If this is what happens with a 50 percent coinsurance rate, imagine what happens with standard coinsurance products that require consumers to pay a fixed amount or cost percentage on the order of 20 percent or $25. In that situation, the profit-maximizing price would be even higher. To prevent this, most insurance companies include rules and constraints that try to influence this price elasticity of demand—the price sensitivity. From the standpoint of pharmaceutical manufacturers, determining the market price sensitivity can be difficult

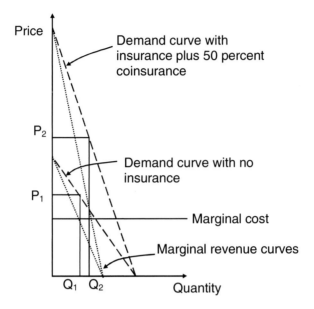

FIGURE 5-1 Representative consumer demand curves for medical care with no insurance coverage compared to coverage with 50 percent coinsurance.
SOURCE: Danzon presentation, February 9, 2009.

because they have essentially three consumers to serve: the patient, the payor, and the physician.

Pricing Incentives for Pharmacy- and Physician-Dispensed Drugs

Different pricing incentives operate for drugs that are dispensed by physicians, which include most oncology products, compared to those that are dispensed by pharmacies free from any physician stake in dispensing. Pharmacy-dispensed drugs are generally handled through pharmacy benefit managers (PBMs) similar to the Medicare part D prescription drug plans or tiered formularies in private payor systems. In essence, these systems establish drug formularies with the lowest tier and co-pay for generics and higher tiers for branded drugs. By tiering the drugs with differences in co-pays, the PBM has a lever to negotiate discounts with the manufacturer. If a drug is placed on a tier with a lower co-pay, then the manufacturer can expect to get a bigger share of the market, and manufacturers are willing to give discounts in return for this preferred formulary status. This mechanism of negotiating discounts through the PBM works reasonably well in therapeutic categories containing several drugs that can be substituted for one another and where patients and physicians have no strong preference between them. However, the mechanism works much less well for cancer drugs that cannot easily be substituted for one another and where physicians and patients want greater freedom of choice. In practice, many plans place cancer drugs on a third or fourth tier, and patients are expected to pay a percentage of the cost through coinsurance.

Physician-dispensed drugs, including many oncology products, are generally covered by Medicare part B or by private insurance through the patient's medical benefit. For these drugs, the physician's reimbursement plays a key role in pricing decisions, and perhaps in dispensing decisions. Before 2005, Medicare reimbursed physicians 95 percent of the Average Wholesale Price (AWP), which is a list price, and pharmaceutical firms discounted this list price to physicians to gain market share while increasing physician margins. In this situation, there was little constraint on the AWP. In 2006, when Medicare began to reimburse based on the Average Sales Price (ASP) plus a 6 percent dispensing fee, no constraint was put on the cost that determined Medicare reimbursement, and the 6 percent fee created perverse incentives to dispense more expensive drugs because these drugs increased physician reimbursement and margin. The absence of a constraint on ASP, combined with the perverse competitive effect of the 6 percent margin, creates an incentive structure that may drive prices up.

Given the stop-loss measures in place in Medicare part D and private plans, plus the supplementary coverage (Medigap or Medicaid) to aid patients in paying the 20 percent co-pay for Medicare part B drugs, the degree of constraint on manufacturers' cancer drug pricing by patient cost sharing is unclear. Medicare part B rules create very little incentive for manufacturers to compete by lowering prices, and the prices set by part B likely spill over into those for part D because manufacturers launching products into both markets tend to make the prices comparable. Overall, this system appears to include few incentives for manufacturers to lower prices, Dr. Danzon said.

Comparing Oncology Drug Prices to Other Areas of Medicine: Are They More Expensive?

Comparing prices for cancer drugs with those for other diseases requires a common, standardized health outcome measure and consistent adjustments for relative cost offsets. Cost per quality-adjusted life-year (QALY) gained is the most widely used metric, but cost per QALY is not systematically estimated or published in the United States for medical treatments. Given that this data is not available for drugs in the United States, Dr. Danzon displayed data from an international source, the Canadian Coordinated Drug Review Center (Table 5-1), which is a review body in the Canadian federal government that issues recommendations regarding whether or not drugs should be reimbursed under provincial drug plans based in part on cost-effectiveness. In this dataset the maximum cost per QALY was higher for noncancer drugs, but the median and minimum costs per QALY were higher for the cancer drugs (Table 5-1). For some drugs, data on cost per QALY were not reported. Based on the percentage of these drugs that received a recommendation of "do not list" for reimbursement—60 percent (3 of 5) for cancer and roughly 50 percent (39 of 80) for noncancer—it can tentatively be inferred that a greater percentage of cancer drugs had a higher cost per QALY, either due to higher prices or lower effectiveness, or due to the outright absence of effectiveness data. This is a very small sample and conclusions are therefore very tentative, but taken at face value this provides some evidence, however weak, for higher prices in cancer drugs compared to drugs in other medical fields.

Dr. Danzon explained that data on drug costs per QALY are not systematically available in the United States. Without this data on drugs in the

TABLE 5-1 Canadian Coordinated Drug Review (CCDR) of Cancer Versus Noncancer Drugs

	Cancer Treatments	Noncancer Treatments
Number of drug indications reviewed	10	100
Number of drugs with cost/QALY reported	5	20
Maximum cost/QALY	$126,500	$363,516
Mean cost/QALY	$73,900	$78,099
Median cost/QALY	$71,000	$61,000
Minimum cost/QALY	$36,000	$9,225
CCDR recommendation		
Do not list for reimbursement	2	8
Number of drugs without cost/QALY reported	5	80
CCDR recommendation		
Do not list for reimbursement	3	39

SOURCES: Danzon presentation, February 9, 2009; Canadian Coordinated Drug Review Center; data from May 2004 through December 2008.

United States, can one be sure the Canadian drug prices given above are reasonably similar to those in the United States? For expensive biologics, including cancer therapies, Dr. Danzon said, price indices for some countries suggest that average prices are similar to or higher than those in the United States. However, the variation in prices across major industrialized countries is not large (Figure 5-2). When the prices are normalized by differences in average per-capita income, again most foreign countries' prices for biologics are similar to or higher than those in the United States (Figure 5-3). This argues against the idea that we pay disproportionately higher prices in the United States for biologics compared to other countries. However, drugs in categories other than biologics tend to be priced 30 to 40 percent lower in most European countries, Dr. Danzon added.

In summary, Dr. Danzon said that data simply does not exist to enable valid comparison of prices for United States cancer drugs relative to prices of drugs for other therapies, and this makes it hard for researchers, payors, patients, and physicians to allocate resources efficiently. Data from the Canadian Coordinated Drug Review Center provides some evidence, however weak, that cancer drugs are higher priced than others. U.S. insurance

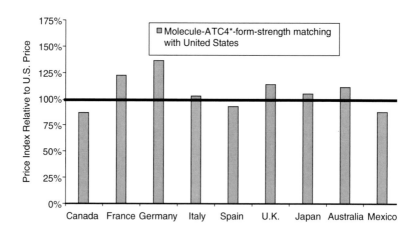

FIGURE 5-2 Biopharmaceutical drug price indices relative to the United States (100 percent level), all biologics including cancer drugs.
NOTE: Calculations based on IMS Health, Inc., MIDAS data, 2005.
* ATC4 = anatomical therapeutic classification, indicates the chemical, therapeutic, and pharmacological subgroup.
SOURCES: Danzon presentation, February 9, 2009; Danzon and Furukawa, 2008.

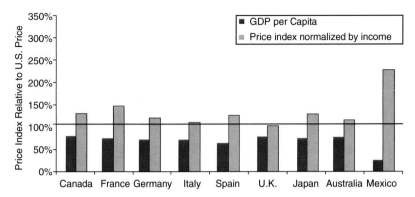

FIGURE 5-3 Biopharmaceutical drug price indices normalized by GDP per capita relative to the United States (100 percent level), all biologics including cancer drugs.
NOTE: Calculations based on IMS Health, Inc., MIDAS data, 2005.
SOURCES: Danzon presentation, February 9, 2009; Danzon and Furukawa, 2008.

reimbursement rules and incentives for physician-dispensed drugs, including many for cancer, may contribute to higher prices. Ultimately, improving the evidence for cost-effectiveness, measured as price per a standardized unit of outcome, will be very important for improving medical care, as well as investment in research and development.

INDUSTRY PERSPECTIVE ON PHARMACEUTICAL PRICING IN ONCOLOGY

Pharmaceutical manufacturers face many challenges inherent in the valuation of cancer products, said Dr. Greg Rossi of Genentech, and the costs of development of cancer therapies can also be quite high. For Avastin (bevacizumab), the cost associated with the development of this product has been roughly $2.5 billion to generate evidence to understand its potential value. With costs and investments such as these, and the risks of not realizing a return on such investments, valuation of therapies, rewarding innovation, and conceptualizing patient-level and societal-level economics for cancer treatments can all be challenging. In addition, the current payment system, which pays for procedures and products but not for quality or outcomes, may be too blunt an instrument than the complexity of cancer requires. How can a more dynamic, nuanced approach to payment policy be created that enables a greater effect on patient outcomes?

Describing Value from the Manufacturer Perspective

There are a large number of factors that influence the manufacturer's price and value of a therapy, and these factors are differentially weighted. They may be differentially weighted depending on the stakeholder (patient, physician, or payor) or depending upon the region. In the United States cancer pharmaceutical marketplace, there is little price elasticity, so formal price elasticity tends not to be the main factor that Genentech considers to determine the price of a product. What Genentech does weight more heavily are various clinical and economic factors, such as the magnitude of the net health benefits in the initial launch indication, the level of unmet need, whether the drug will be introduced as second- or third-line therapy into patient populations that have limited treatment choices, and the potential value in future indications. In many cases, surrogate endpoint data (e.g., response rate) is often all that is known at the time of initial launch in highly refractory disease settings. Therefore, the clinical benefits known at this time may not reflect the full potential value or benefit of a drug for all of its potential indications; for example, whether the therapy has health benefits as frontline treatment for metastatic disease or as adjuvant therapy for one or more cancer type. Genentech performs a number of economic analyses to assess the impact of the new product introduction from a variety of perspectives (patient, provider, managed care plan, and CMS, among others) to determine its value. These analyses include formal cost-effectiveness analyses, budget-impact analyses (perhaps the most important factor for many private managed care organizations in the United States), and out-of-pocket costs for patients to inform both the assessment of product value and some of the practical aspects of a new product introduction.

The factors that influence the value of a treatment vary by stakeholder (Figure 5-4). For regulators such as the FDA, trial data with specific endpoints relative to a highly valid internal control, such as placebo, will be the principal measure of a treatment's benefit, but costs will not factor into their considerations of risks and benefits. For patients and physicians, out-of-pocket costs, adherence, and trial data are of critical importance, as well as things that are not traditionally measured in registration programs, such as treatment impacts on hope for survival and the level of innovation. In addition, physicians and patients are interested in how trial data for a new treatment compares to standard treatments already used in practice. For commercial payors, net price, cost offsets, and data on the treatment from trials in the real world are especially important (Figure 5-4). How should

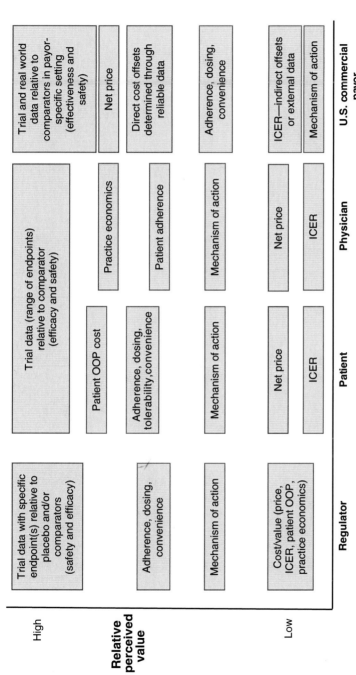

FIGURE 5-4 Measures of relative perceived value by stakeholder or user.

NOTE: ICER = incremental cost-effectiveness ratio; OOP = out-of-pocket (costs).

SOURCE: Rossi presentation, February 9, 2009.

pharmaceutical manufacturers weigh the factors important to these different customers to determine the value of a new treatment at launch?

Dr. Rossi made a few comments on costs. The incremental cost-effectiveness ratio (ICER) is not often used to discuss cost in the United States, he said. Furthermore, when physicians are surveyed on the costs of certain therapies, even common ones, there is high variability in the responses given, perhaps because many physicians do not know the precise costs of their therapies. Differences in patient out-of-pocket costs do not necessarily correlate with differences in the actual price of potential drugs to treat a particular condition because of benefit design. These gaps in knowledge of drug prices further complicate communication between physicians and patients around costs.

From these complications around costs and the complexity around drug benefits to these various stakeholders, can the true costs and benefits of a treatment be precisely identified to determine its value? For total costs, Dr. Rossi said that this may be possible. However, cost data collected in randomized controlled trials (RCTs) may not be predictive of costs in the real world, though they do allow for reasonable cost approximation at either the patient or societal level. For treatment benefits, standard, agreed-upon methods for adjustment of quantity of life are needed to account for quality of that extended life. Cancer trials have focused on the endpoint of quantity of life gained, but we are seeing that overall survival will be more and more challenging to routinely use as an endpoint in many large randomized phase III trials because of a number of factors, most importantly the complexity of follow-on treatments and crossover trial designs.

Figure 5-5 shows the results of an informal analysis of studies from Dr. Rossi's organization of treatments for breast, colorectal, and lung cancer over the last 10 years. This analysis examines the relationship between progression-free survival and overall survival in these studies.

Trials of treatments for metastatic or advanced disease between 1998 and 2008 with at least 100 patients were included in the analysis. Single-arm, single-center, and diagnostic studies were excluded. The 20 largest studies were selected for each of the three cancer types, and the differences in median progression-free survival between the treatment and control arms for each trial were plotted against the median differences in overall survival. The charts show that, compared to control groups in these studies, effects on progression free survival in the intervention groups had a poor predictive value for effects on overall survival in recent breast cancer trials, but had a better predictive value in studies of colon cancer and non-small-cell

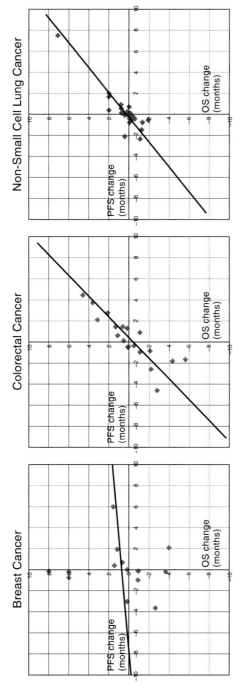

FIGURE 5-5 Relationship between differences in median progression-free survival and overall survival in treatment versus control arms from studies of breast, colorectal, and lung cancer treatments.

NOTE: Each plot includes the 20 largest studies meeting inclusion and exclusion criteria for each tumor type between 1998 and 2008. Inclusion criteria: trials with progression-free survival and overall survival as endpoints, English language studies between 1998 and 2008, and 100 or more patients with metastatic or advanced disease. Exclusion criteria: single-arm, single-center, and diagnostic studies.

NOTE: OS = overall survival; PFS = progression-free survival. Differences in region, year trial was conducted, crossover design, population risk factors, subsequent therapies, and quality of the trials need to be considered but are not captured by the graphs.

SOURCES: Rossi presentation, February 9, 2009; Genentech, Inc. study data, 1998–2008.

lung cancer trials (Figure 5-5). A challenge to the research and clinical communities trying to understand value, Dr. Rossi explained, is finding other surrogate endpoints to better approximate definitive clinical endpoints and what outcome heterogeneity exists across the patient subgroups within a certain patient population.

Dr. Rossi proposed that there may be different, nonsurvival outcomes worth considering. For first-line therapy, certain outcomes could be characterized based on symptomatology, toxicity or tolerability, convenience, other health-related quality of life, emotional domains, physical function, activities of daily living, productivity, or economic costs. Some studies have successfully characterized such outcomes as these for a particular line of therapy, such as for Tarceva in lung cancer or Sutent in renal cell carcinoma gathered by Pfizer and their clinical collaborators. However, beyond changes in these domains as the disease progresses and treatment changes (i.e., differences in pre- and post-progression health states), what other endpoints can be incorporated to characterize the value of a treatment to patients? The data on endpoints after progression are sparse but deserve greater attention.

Patient-reported outcomes are also often excluded from clinical trials in cancer. Michael Woolley and colleagues examined all industry-sponsored studies listed at www.clinicaltrials.gov in the cancer domain for whether or not they included patient-reported primary or secondary endpoints, as well as whether or not patient-reported outcomes and symptoms were included in the specific labels of new cancer therapies (Gondek et al., 2007). Overall, of 2,704 oncology trials listed, only 322 (12 percent) included a patient-reported outcome measure, and only 6 (9 percent) of 70 FDA new or revised labels included patient-reported data. Dr. Rossi saw this as a call to action for patient-reported outcomes, saying, "If we believe them to be valuable, we had better start measuring them, and we had better be able to talk about them."

Dynamic Value and Pricing for Oncology Drugs

In the pharmaceutical industry, the dynamic value of a drug depends upon its different value propositions for different lines of therapy in different diseases. Dynamic value is particularly important to consider in cancer therapy because cancer products are built with multiple indications—front line, second line, breast cancer, lung cancer, adjuvant therapy, and so on—each with different implications for a drug's value. In the case of Herceptin (trastuzumab), the drug was launched into a specific patient population in

1998 as frontline therapy for metastatic breast cancer. It showed a significant median overall survival improvement of 4.8 months, and its cost per QALY was over $100,000 (Elkin et al., 2004). This was significantly higher than the cost-effectiveness thresholds established in many countries. In the adjuvant phase, trastuzumab has subsequently been shown to have a much lower cost per QALY of $26,400 (Garrison et al., 2007). But the opportunity to test trastuzumab in the adjuvant breast cancer setting was predicated on its approval for use in the metastatic phase. If Genentech were to price trastuzumab according to a cost-effectiveness threshold, one might argue that the price should be discounted significantly for the treatment of metastatic breast cancer and increased substantially for adjuvant treatment. The case of Avastin (bevacizumab) was even more complicated. At the time of launch, Dr. Rossi explained, bevacizumab had failed a phase III trial for treatment of breast cancer, shown significant impact in colorectal cancer, and further studies were underway for treatment of lung cancer. What should the price have been based on? The first indication? The average effect over the life cycle? Weighting for endpoint or disease severity? It was decided that pricing of bevacizumab would be based on its benefits and costs compared to analogues for the same indications, such as Erbitux, irinotecan, and oxaliplatin, which had also recently launched. When it became clear through phase III studies in breast and lung cancer indications that bevacizumab optimally benefited patients at a higher dose in these settings, the Avastin patient-assistance program was put into place so that patients who required more than 10,000 milligrams of the drug could subsequently receive it at no further cost. There have been no price increases since that time. These examples raise important questions. As we think about value-based pricing of pharmaceuticals, how can the complexity of a product's indications and life cycle be taken into account for initial pricing? How willing are we to pay for innovations, especially for "first-in-class" therapy innovations that can pave the way for other therapies and biosimilars, generate evidence of success in therapeutic approach, further knowledge of appropriate patient populations through biomarker and subgroup identification, and may lead to reduced costs of subsequent therapies in their class through the development of biosimilars?

In closing, Dr. Rossi said that he expected better outcomes in cancer care to be achieved through combining targeted therapies in specific patient subgroups. How patient benefit is defined and measured to determine value will be critical to understand and incorporate ahead of time in the development of future therapeutics and companion diagnostics studies. Managing costs while enhancing value will include both pricing-related and nonpricing-related steps. Nonpricing steps could include using companion diagnostics to identify responders to treatment, considering patient-reported outcomes in measures of treatment benefit, integrating economic evaluations into study design, enhancing patient-assistance programs, and generating evidence after launch to understand real-world outcomes. Pricing steps could include expenditure caps and patient risk sharing. Ultimately, we will have to be innovative both in terms of advances in cancer treatments and in terms of oncology payment policy.

BUILDING THE EVIDENCE BASE FOR VALUE OF NEW TREATMENTS: COST-EFFECTIVENESS ANALYSES ALONGSIDE CANCER CLINICAL TRIALS

Cancer care providers include a wide variety of health care professionals in collaboration, particularly in the area of cancer clinical research. As a clinician and a clinical researcher, Dr. Deborah Schrag of the Dana-Farber Cancer Institute recognized the obligation those in her position had to promote value from a number of different perspectives. Patient needs—survival, hope, trust, compassion, access, and recognition of personhood—had to be reconciled with research obligations to society at large and considerations of cost-effectiveness, cost-utility, efficiency, and equity in the distribution of resources. These sets of obligations are layered onto the unique concerns of oncology providers themselves, including their interest in respect, professionalism, and security. Economic security in particular is often difficult for providers to talk about. For clinical researchers, balancing multiple perspectives and the obligations that accompany them can be challenging.

Creating Value and Understanding Costs in Clinical Trials

Individual physicians make hundreds of risk and benefit calculations for individual patients on a daily basis, taking into account their knowledge of the literature, their previous experience with other patients, their judgment about the individuals they treat, and the preferences they and their patients hold. With all of these factors to consider, how can medical oncologists systematically determine treatment value with respect to cost in the context of clinical trials? A systematic approach that is relatively little-used in the United States is cost-effectiveness analysis. Cost-effectiveness analyses are comparisons that can take the form of

- Cost-minimization analysis to determine which treatment costs more: treatment A or treatment B;

- Cost-effectiveness analysis with units of life-years gained; or
- Cost-utility analysis with units of quality-adjusted or quality-discounted life-years, which can also be expressed in terms of the incremental cost-effectiveness ratio (ICER).

The latter is the optimal approach, but estimation of the ICER requires that one treatment strategy be compared to an alternative. Sometimes the alternative is no treatment, but more often it is the default treatment standard.

Cost-effectiveness analyses are useful when both the efficacy and the cost of a treatment are greater than those of the standard of care. In trials, cost-effectiveness analyses are most needed when the treatment benefit is small but affects a large population, when a new treatment is particularly costly compared to standard treatment, or when there is simply a high degree of uncertainty regarding the economic effect of a new treatment. Typically these analyses are considered in later-stage (i.e., phase III) trials once the probability of a drug reaching market is higher. Given the resources required to estimate cost effectiveness, and that comparison of two alternative strategies is essential, cost-effectiveness analysis does not make sense in the context of phase I or II studies.

Ideally, cost-effectiveness analyses are built into the trial with clear specification of data-collection and analytic methods, and data is gathered prospectively. However, preliminary data (e.g., power calculations for cost-effectiveness analyses) to inform data-collection methods may be absent, meaning that post hoc analytic plans are often applied to prospective data. Retrospective data assembly may be used once a treatment has shown clinical efficacy, tallying resource utilization post hoc from either the original study population or a comparable one.

Given the complexity and intensive resources required to integrate cost-effectiveness analyses into phase III clinical trials, back-of-the-envelope calculations are often used to identify key cost drivers (see Box 5-1). Such calculations are fast, inexpensive, and potentially misleading, particularly when they rely on assembly of retrospective data that were not collected for this purpose. Often key cost drivers are unavailable.

Challenges in Conducting Cost-Effectiveness Analyses in Cancer Trials

There are immense challenges in conducting cost-effectiveness analyses in cancer clinical trials. To illustrate this point, Dr. Schrag presented data

---

BOX 5-1
Back-of-the-Envelope Cost-Effectiveness Analysis:
What Is the Incremental Benefit of Adding Erlotinib
to Gemcitabine for Pancreatic Cancer?

Overall survival benefit	12.8 days
Quality-adjusted survival assuming mild erlotinib toxicities—most frequently diarrhea, rash	9.4 days
Quality-adjusted survival assuming severe erlotinib toxicity—most frequently diarrhea, rash	8 days
Lifetime incremental costs per patient:	
Costs of erlotinib	$10,300
Costs of adverse events	$780
Costs of extra survival time	$4,100
Total costs	$15,200
Costs per life-year (costs of erlotinib plus costs of extra survival time all divided by years of overall survival gained)	$410,000
Costs per QALY (adjusted for mild to severe symptoms)	$430,000 (mild) to $510,000 (severe)

SOURCE: Schrag presentation, February 9, 2009; adapted from Miksad et al., 2007.

---

from a cost-effectiveness analysis, the COST study (Nelson et al., 2004), performed as part of a phase III cooperative group RCT in which the two study arms—laparoscopic-assisted colectomy versus open colectomy to treat resectable colon cancer—showed similar patient quality of life, cancer recurrence rate, survival, and complications (Clinical Outcomes of Surgical Therapy Study Group, 2004; Weeks et al., 2002). With such similar outcomes, it made sense to look at differences in cost, and a cost-minimization analysis was performed to answer the question of whether laparoscopic-assisted colectomy was less expensive than open colectomy. The study took the perspective of a third-party payor, and an intention-to-treat analysis was performed, as would be the case in any clinical trial. The time horizon used has important implications for any cost-effectiveness analysis, and the study investigators chose a 2-month postoperative horizon after making sure that there were no treatment differences in late outcomes. Hospital costs vary geographically and by hospital, so standard cost-effectiveness analysis methodology is to measure resource utilization, itemize all the services and equipment likely to differ between the study arms, and then convert this to standard unit costs. In this study, patients who had open colectomy stayed in the hospital 1.2 days longer, but the laparoscopy-assisted colectomy patients spent an average of 57 more minutes in the operating room where a greater number of surgical equipment cartridges were used (see Table 5-2). Unit costs were difficult to obtain and varied between academic and community hospitals. At academic centers, a hospital day costs almost 50 percent more than at community hospitals, but the cost of operating room professionals was less. Therefore, the result of the cost comparison between the two arms depends on whether academic or community hospital unit costs apply (see Table 5-3). As a result of running

TABLE 5-2 Resources Used by Colectomy Method—Laparoscopic-Assisted vs. Open

| | Colectomy Method | | |
Resource Category	Laparoscopic-Assisted	Open	*P*-Value
Mean length of stay, days	5.5	6.7	< .001
Mean operating room time, minutes	166	109	< .001
Equipment cartridges used per patient	3.4	2.5	< .001

SOURCES: Schrag presentation, February 9, 2009; Clinical Outcomes of Surgical Therapy Study Group, 2004.

TABLE 5-3 Cost of Resources Used by Colectomy Method, at Academic and Community Hospitals

| | Cost (2007 $US) | |
Resource Category	Academic Center	Community Hospital
Hospital day	1,426	925
Laparoscopic-assisted colectomy: professional component of surgery	1,676	2,105
Open colectomy: professional component of surgery	1,653	2,065
Laparoscopic-assisted colectomy: technical component of surgery plus fixed operating room supplies	3,454	5,472
Open colectomy: technical component of surgery plus fixed operating room supplies	3,204	3,738

SOURCES: Schrag presentation, February 9, 2009; Clinical Outcomes of Surgical Therapy Study Group, 2004.

the operating room longer and with higher personnel costs at the community hospitals, laparoscopic-assisted colectomy cost $2,454 more at community hospitals compared to open colectomy while saving $62 at academic centers (see Table 5-4).

What were the lessons learned from this study? Economically, the choice between laparoscopic-assisted and open colectomy consists of a trade-off between higher operative costs and shorter hospital length of stay. Laparoscopic-assisted colectomy is relatively less expensive at institutions with higher rooming but lower operative personnel costs. Taking the true opportunity cost of community surgeons' time into account, however, this operative approach will actually be more expensive in most settings.

Companion cost-effectiveness analyses such as these are challenging. If the primary study fails to meet its clinical endpoint, the cost-effectiveness analysis is rendered moot and uninteresting. For instance, one cost-effectiveness companion to an RCT comparing gemcitabine plus bevacizumab to gemcitabine plus placebo for pancreatic cancer was stopped after 2 years of intensive data collection when bevacizumab was found to provide no additional benefit. Another example, an ongoing companion to a large RCT for colorectal cancer, has been modified multiple times to keep up with study design changes to reflect new first-line therapies and the addition of KRAS biomarker testing for patients on cetuximab. Ultimately, these studies can be useful, but they have all the risks and caveats of

TABLE 5-4 Incremental Unit Costs by Colectomy Method at Academic and Community Hospitals

	Incremental Cost of Laparoscopic-Assisted Colectomy (2007 $US)	
	Unit Costs from Academic Center	Unit Costs from Community Hospital
Hospital stay cost	−1,665	−1,083
Operating room total cost	1,142	3,275
Anesthesia total cost	89	140
Recovery	10	−16
Intensive care unit days	659	333
Reoperation	−2	−1
Rehospitalization	−293	−189
TOTAL	−62	2,454

SOURCES: Schrag presentation, February 9, 2009; data obtained courtesy of Dr. Jane Weeks; Clinical Outcomes of Surgical Therapy Study Group, 2004.

the trials they accompany. It is also exceedingly difficult to secure funding for cost-effectiveness analyses in the United States. Cost-effectiveness data cannot be explicitly considered when coverage decisions are made and this undoubtedly helps to explain the difficulty obtaining funding to support these studies.

Patient Concerns Over the Cost of Prescription Drugs

Even if oncologists were able to understand a treatment's cost-effectiveness, would it matter to patients? Or are cancer patients insensitive to treatment costs when making treatment decisions? How much do patients worry about the costs of their treatments? Do they discuss these concerns with providers on their oncology team? Dr. Schrag presented preliminary results from a survey she and her colleagues performed involving 409 patients who were asked these questions. Thirty-nine percent were not worried, 31 percent were a little worried, and only 10 percent were very worried about the costs of treatment. Among those who were very worried about the costs of treatment, 77 percent of them had not discussed these concerns with their doctors. Clearly, most patients are much more worried about their cancer and their symptoms than they are about costs, Dr. Schrag said. But in cases where patients have significant cost concerns, much more discussion is needed with doctors.

To summarize, Dr. Schrag listed barriers to integration of cost-effectiveness analyses in evaluation of cancer treatment. These barriers include

- Substantial data-collection efforts are required to obtain reliable data,
- Lack of data systems architecture in place to support cost-effectiveness analyses,
- Reluctance of institutions to share cost data,
- Investigator suspicion of the validity of cost-effectiveness analyses,
- Underdeveloped cost-effectiveness analytic methods,
- Competing study priorities and limited funding,
- Occasional irrelevance of the cost-effectiveness analyses' results,
- Political and regulatory hurdles mean the information cannot be used in regulatory decisions, and
- Cultural preferences to avoid cost-effectiveness analyses for fear of "rationing."

Dr. Schrag concluded that a variety of strategies to build the evidence base are needed to increase value in oncology. More and better information is always needed on what works, how clinicians treat, and the consequences. We will need to accept limitations and coverage restrictions that will curb the use of expensive treatment technologies in circumstances where there really is no supporting evidence, she said. On the horizon of a new era of personalized medicine, what is going to be funded—cost-effectiveness analyses or the development of more biomarkers? Can we fund both?

DISCUSSION

Dr. Lee Newcomer of UnitedHealthcare asked Dr. Rossi why the Avastin patient-assistance program appeared to be underutilized. Dr. Rossi replied that the underuse was caused by the program not being actively promoted by the company.

Dr. Bhadrasain Vikram of the National Cancer Institute asked Dr. Rossi what Genentech's strategy was for collecting real-world outcomes. Dr. Rossi replied that, while RCTs remain the cornerstone of evidence development, Genentech had just begun a disease-based registry in breast cancer to look at patterns of care, health economics, patient-reported outcomes, and clinical outcomes in the real world.

Dr. Allen Lichter of the American Society of Clinical Oncology asked Dr. Schrag whether there were ways to anticipate at the outset the study population size needed to definitely achieve a cost-effectiveness trial result—similar to power calculations for trials of clinical benefit. She said that techniques such as adaptive trial design, dynamic trial design, and value-of-information theory could be used to calculate such a threshold ahead of time, but the crucial component is also to understand key cost drivers, which can be difficult before the trial has begun.

Dr. Thomas Smith of the Virginia Commonwealth University Massey Cancer Center pointed out two examples of competitor drugs increasing the price of all the drugs in a market after they were introduced—aromatase inhibitors in breast cancer and thalidomide derivatives. How can market forces improve the drug prices that patients pay? Dr. Rossi responded by saying that this was an area for comparative effectiveness research to show true drug equivalency and support direct competition. He also noted markets where the introduction of competitor drugs have reduced prices.

Dr. Smith commented from his experience that it was especially hard for patients in safety net health centers to afford their anticancer treatments. Often enrollment in pharmaceutical manufacturers' indigent care programs is spectacularly difficult and complex. These barriers prevented many disadvantaged patients from being able to benefit from modern chemotherapeutic drugs they needed.

Dr. Jane Perlmutter of the Gemini Group asked why the value of a patient's time had not been factored in the cost-effectiveness analysis example Dr. Schrag showed in detail. Dr. Schrag acknowledged that this could be an important consideration in some studies and that significant literature exists on ways to collect information from patients on their time costs.

Dr. Lerner asked whether the current economic situation had put a greater pressure on patients and doctors to discuss price, since more patients are in economic distress. Dr. Schrag thought that this was the case. Patients do not have employment security anymore, she said, and employers in this economy can be forced to lay off even employees with new cancer diagnoses. Physicians have come to rely on social workers and legal assistance for patients more often and earlier for people in jeopardy. Some patients want to talk about costs very directly, but they are a small minority. Most decide not to think about it. Just like the mortgage market was unsustainable, this avoidance of the cost issue is equally unsustainable.

REFERENCES

Clinical Outcomes of Surgical Therapy Study Group. 2004. A comparison of laparoscopically assisted and open colectomy for colon cancer. *New England Journal of Medicine* 350(20):2050–2059.

Danzon, P. M., and M. F. Furukawa. 2008. International prices and availability of pharmaceuticals in 2005. *Health Affairs* 27(1):221–233.

Elkin, E. B., M. C. Weinstein, E. P. Winer, K. M. Kunitz, S. J. Schnitt, and J. C. Weeks. 2004. HER-2 testing and trastuzumab therapy for metastatic breast cancer: A cost-effectiveness analysis. *Journal of Clinical Oncology* 22(5):854–863.

Garrison, L. P., D. Lubeck, D. Lalla, V. Paton, A. Dueck, and E. A. Perez. 2007. Cost-effectiveness analysis of trastuzumab in the adjuvant setting for treatment of HER2-positive breast cancer. *Cancer* 110(3):489–498.

Gondek, K., P.-P. Sagnier, K. Gilchrist, and J. M. Woolley. 2007. Current status of patient-reported outcomes in industry-sponsored oncology trials and product labels. *Journal of Clinical Oncology* 25(32):5087–5093.

Miksad, R. A., L. Schnipper, and M. Goldstein. 2007. Does a statistically significant survival benefit of erlotinib plus gemcitabine for advanced pancreatic cancer translate into clinical significance and value? *Journal of Clinical Oncology* 25(28):4506–4507.

Weeks, J. C., H. Nelson, S. Gelber, D. Sargent, G. Schroeder, and for the Clinical Outcomes of Surgical Therapy (COST) Study Group. 2002. Short-term quality-of-life outcomes following laparoscopic-assisted colectomy vs. open colectomy for colon cancer. *Journal of the American Medical Association* 287(3):321–328.

6

Value in Oncology Practice: Oncologist and Health Insurer Perspectives

ONCOLOGISTS' PERCEPTION OF VALUE

Dr. Peter Neumann of Tufts Medical Center explained that his group at the Center for Evaluation of Value and Risk in Health at the Tufts Institute for Clinical Research and Health Policy Studies was interested in how people used—or perhaps did not use—cost-effectiveness information, how it is communicated, and how it is perceived. The cost-effectiveness literature contains numerous studies in oncology. In 2006, roughly 260 studies that examined cost per quality-adjusted life-year (QALY) were published in the cost-utility literature, and about 30 had applications in oncology (CEVR, 2009). In the literature containing cost-per-life-year studies and similar endpoints outside of oncology, the number is orders of magnitude larger. Many of these studies are in leading medical journals that are widely read by physicians. This raises a question: who is using all of these data, and to what extent are oncologists influenced by costs in their treatment recommendations?

To answer this question, Dr. Neumann, along with Eric Nadler and Benjamin Eckert (Nadler et al., 2006), published a study of 90 oncologists from two leading academic medical centers who responded to a series of survey prompts regarding their views on costs and cost-effectiveness in cancer treatment. The study found that 77.5 percent of oncologists studied agreed that every patient should have access to effective cancer treatments regardless of their costs. Far fewer, only 30 percent, agreed that the costs of new cancer drugs currently influence their decisions. Eighty-one percent agreed that patient out-of-pocket therapy costs influence their decisions, and a similar majority agreed that the costs of new cancer drugs would impose greater rationing in oncology in the next 5 years (Nadler et al., 2006). These answers seem to reveal a somewhat conflicted relationship with treatment costs among these oncologists, reflecting some of the challenges that oncologists currently face.

The same study posed a series of hypothetical scenarios to the oncologists surveyed. They were first asked to "Imagine a new cancer medication for treatment of metastatic lung cancer that on average costs $70,000 more than standard of care. At what minimum improvement in overall survival would you prescribe the new medication instead of the standard of care?" The distribution of responses is shown in Figure 6-1. Even though most surveyed oncologists agreed that costs should not affect care decisions, a majority required a minimum 2–4 months added survival to warrant the $70,000 expense. But there were a few at the extremes, such as one oncologist who would prescribe the medication for just one day of added survival. From the average minimum survival benefit required by these oncologists, Neumann and Nadler derived a mean cost-effectiveness threshold implied by the oncologists' responses—$318,000 per life-year gained (Nadler et al., 2006). The authors concluded that oncologists' cost-effectiveness threshold

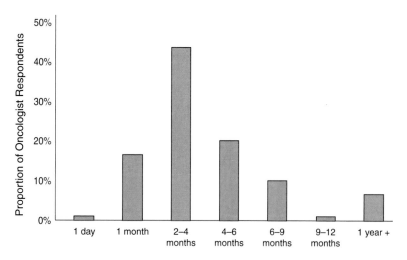

FIGURE 6-1 Distribution of oncologist responses: hypothetical survival benefit needed to justify a treatment expense of $70,000.
SOURCES: Neumann presentation, February 9, 2009; Nadler et al., 2006.

for new cancer therapies seem to be high, at least compared to conventional health care cost-effectiveness thresholds. At the same time, oncologists were not sure whether expensive new therapies offer good value. After selecting their minimum survival benefit for an incremental cost of $70,000, the oncologists were asked "Do you think that reflects good value?" Most said it did not.

Dr. Neumann explained that he and his colleagues are completing a follow-up study to determine the extent to which oncologists nationwide believe that costs influence their prescribing behavior, whether they discuss costs with patients, and how they feel about various reimbursement policies.

Dr. Neumann concluded that costs seem to influence oncologists' treatment recommendations, oncologists do not seem to communicate frequently about costs with their patients, oncologists seem to favor cost-effectiveness information while wanting to remain in charge of their own decisions. There also appears to be some enthusiasm among oncologists for price controls, but most did not favor more cost sharing on the part of patients. Clearly, costs are a central concern in health care today and there is a need for better communication between physicians and patients.

PAYING FOR NEW CANCER TREATMENTS: RIGHTS AND RESPONSIBILITIES OF HEALTH INSURERS

Ever since Benjamin Franklin opened the first fire insurance company, explained Dr. Newcomer, the responsibility of the insurer has been to spread risk among a group of people and save them from catastrophic financial distress. Payors in health care do the same thing: they pool funds among groups of people so that, when an individual member gets sick, he or she can pay to treat the illness. Insurers also have a responsibility to maintain a capital pool that has fiscal integrity. During the 1980s, insurers gained a third responsibility—that of negotiating on behalf of their members to find reasonable prices for therapies considered effective. However, the entire health industry has failed in this third responsibility, with premiums for a California family of four increasing from only 15 percent of U.S. minimum wage earnings in 1970 to 101 percent in 2005[1] (GAO, 1975). The system

---

[1] Figures reflect monthly Federal Employees Health Benefits (FEHBP) total premiums for the government-wide Blue Cross/Blue Shield options for non-postal workers and minimum wage earnings for full time work of 173.33 hours per month (2,080 hours per year/12) in California.

is broken, and we are going to need to do something fairly radical to change it, Dr. Newcomer said.

Health insurers, or payors, look at value very differently than one would for FDA studies or phase III randomized controlled trials (RCTs), as these trials' results are limited to a very tightly defined group of patients in controlled treatments. These trials are not the real world. In the real world, there is what Dr. Newcomer called "the cascade of chaos" during the dissemination of any new therapy to the nation's community health care providers. First, the treatment is approved and promptly used by providers, often with many errors because they lack experience with the treatment. Eventually the errors subside as providers become more familiar with the treatment; they then begin tweaking the indications, and this ultimately leads to large indication extrapolation and off-label usage. The introduction of trastuzumab (Herceptin) for HER2-positive breast cancer was no different. Reddy and colleagues showed that inexperienced community labs misclassified 15 percent of those told they overexpressed the HER2 gene when they actually underexpressed the gene and had no chance of responding to trastuzumab. Conversely, 10 percent of those the community labs said underexpressed the gene actually were overexpressers who should have been treated but were not (Reddy et al., 2006). To make matters worse, when oncologists were asked to document HER2 overexpression in patients receiving trastuzumab, 8 percent of patients being treated showed no evidence of overexpression, and 4 percent of patients on trastuzumab treatment had no genetic test results at all. Combining the laboratory errors and physician misinterpretation of results, the study found over one-third of patients were receiving the wrong treatment due to inexperience. These error rates were caused in large part by inexperience reading and reporting the test results. Before long, oncologists began tweaking the indications for trastuzumab, bending the limits to treat patients whose overexpression tests stained at "2+" strength, rather than strictly those whose result was a "3+" stain. Finally, physicians began to move to off-label uses, such as continuing trastuzumab treatment through multiple relapses and metastases, despite no evidence of efficacy to support these uses (Pusztai and Esteva, 2006). The cascade of chaos has clearly lowered the value of trastuzumab and other therapies like it in the real world.

Inconsistency in Cancer Treatment

Inconsistency in cancer treatments also reduces value in cancer care even for well-established therapies. Dr. Newcomer showed a series of pictograph grids representing the drug, dose, and schedule regimens of patients with metastatic breast cancer from practices reimbursed by UnitedHealthcare. The one thing they had in common was that none of the treatment regimens resembled one another, showing that there was no uniform treatment of metastatic breast cancer in these community settings. Jack Wennberg also showed considerable treatment inconsistency when he studied a Medicare data set to determine health care resources used for patients in the 6 months before they died, comparing the data across the 77 top hospitals listed in *U.S. News and World Report* (Wennberg et al., 2004). There was considerable geographic variation in the number of hospital days and physician visits per patient (Figures 6-2 and 6-3). These data imply that assessments of value in cancer care using clinical evidence from Palo Alto will be markedly different from the same assessment using clinical evidence from Manhattan. As a payor, the geographic area one covers will distort the value obtained for a given service or treatment.

Dr. Newcomer then showed data on inconsistency in cetuximab and panitumumab treatment for metastatic colon cancer among patients with UnitedHealthcare coverage. Inexplicably, patients with identical conditions receiving the same drug had an average of either 5.3 treatment cycles at $4,428 per cycle at outpatient facilities or 9 cycles at $2,693 per cycle when treated in the physician's office. There was no correlation between physician fee schedule and use of the outpatient facilities. Clearly, there is a great deal of inconsistency in adult oncology that hampers assessment of its value.

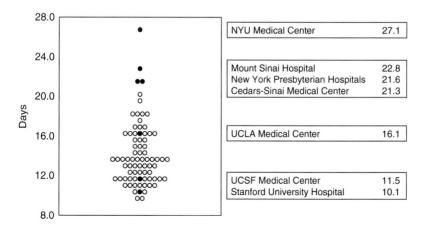

FIGURE 6-2 Days in hospital during the last 6 months of life.
SOURCES: Newcomer presentation, February 9, 2009; Wennberg et al., 2004.

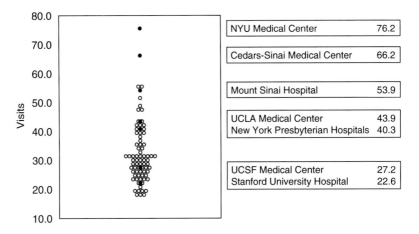

FIGURE 6-3 Average number of physician visits per patient during the last 6 months of life.
SOURCES: Newcomer presentation, February 9, 2009; Wennberg et al., 2004.

Dr. Newcomer's Proposals for Improving Value in Cancer Care

First, Dr. Newcomer said, the United States needs its own National Institute for Health and Clinical Excellence (NICE). Eventually, a certain cost per QALY will have to be set as our cost-effectiveness limit for a treatment, and beyond that we simply cannot cover it in an insurance package. Second, Dr. Newcomer wondered if a new FDA designation of "scientific approval" could be created to require new drugs with uncertain economic benefits to be covered only if the patients receive them in controlled ways with no off-label uses (while enrolled in registries or trials, for example) to build scientific evidence for the drug. The drug would then be reevaluated after 3 years for a final decision. Third, Dr. Newcomer emphasized that consistent practices across providers and geographies had to be achieved. He described work he had begun with medical oncology groups who had decided on their own to go to standardized therapies of their choosing. These groups are going to be incentivized differently for standardizing treatments, explained Dr. Newcomer—they will be paid for patient services rather than based on the drugs they use. UnitedHealthcare plans to observe these practices and compare outcomes of the standardized treatments they choose as a type of cluster randomized study. It is hoped that this will advance best practices faster than RCTs.

In closing, Dr. Newcomer concluded that the way valuation of treatments occurs must be changed. Compact clinical trials that are currently used do not represent the actual value of treatments once they reach the community. The underlying system that assesses value must be changed because the one we have today doesn't work.

INTERNATIONAL PERSPECTIVES ON ASSESSING VALUE FOR ONCOLOGY PRODUCTS

European countries, with all of their variation, differ quite a bit in their use of oncology products, said Michael Drummond of the University of York. Many eastern European countries, with lower gross domestic product (GDP) per capita, are quickly adopting modern medicines to keep pace with the West. The evidence-based medicine approach is common in northern European countries and gaining ground in southern countries. Most European health care systems are based on national health services or social insurance, and hospitals, along with cancer drugs, are funded through global budgets or case mix-related payments. Health technology assessment (HTA) is growing and there are many clinical practice guidelines. Recently, HTA with cost-effectiveness analysis has been used more and more in reimbursement and coverage decisions, with the United Kingdom, Netherlands, Hungary, Belgium, Finland, Norway, Portugal, Sweden, Slovakia, Ireland, and Germany leading this trend while Spain, Italy, and France consider whether or not to follow suit.

Cancer drugs account for 10–15 percent of total cancer care expenditure, and their costs are increasing 15–20 percent per year. With respect to expenditure per capita on cancer drugs of different vintages, the United States shows the highest spending overall and considerable spending on newer drugs while the United Kingdom shows less overall spending and very little spending on new drugs (Figure 6-4). Dr. Drummond showed a series of international comparisons of the uptake of cancer drugs (imatinib, trastuzumab, cetuximab, and bevacizumab). In each comparison the United States led all others in uptake and overall usage of the drugs.

The National Institute for Health and Clinical Excellence (NICE) was created in 1999 as part of the United Kingdom's National Health Service (NHS), and it receives funding from the government. Most physicians do not believe it is independent of the government, and NICE is widely seen as a rationing body because of its health technology appraisal program, though it has programs in other areas such as public health interventions,

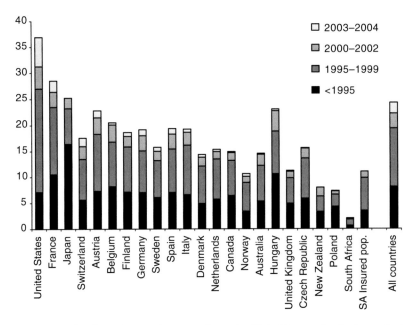

FIGURE 6-4 Adjusted per capita cancer drug sales (€) in 22 countries, by drug-release year (2005 data).
SOURCES: Drummond presentation, February 9, 2009; Jonsson and Wilking, 2007; based on IMS Health, IMS MIDAS Quantum (for South Africa, sales per capita is presented along with two capita rates for the total population as well as for the insured [18.5%] population).

new investigational procedures, and clinical guideline development. Also, the program takes care to appraise both a treatment's clinical effectiveness and its cost-effectiveness. The health technology appraisal program has two tracks:

1. Multiple technology appraisal (MTA) is a full systematic review and economic analysis performed by independent centers (mostly academic) of several drugs in a treatment class or several technologies simultaneously. It requires 54 weeks.
2. Single technology appraisal (STA) was introduced as a fast-track appraisal process. STA is not an independent appraisal but a detailed analysis of a drug company's submitted analysis without external review. It requires 39 weeks. To date, almost all of the drugs that have gone through STA have been cancer treatments.

The health technology appraisal program at NICE has also employed a cost-effectiveness threshold of £20,000 to £30,000 per QALY gained, or roughly $30,000 to $50,000 per QALY (at the time of the workshop), for approval. Above this threshold, drugs are unlikely to be approved for use by the NHS.

Dr. Drummond presented his research on NICE guidance regarding new cancer drugs appraised between May 2000 to March 2008. Data were extracted from published NICE technology appraisals and eventual licensure in the United Kingdom NICE drug appraisal outcomes were classified for each indication at one of three levels: (1) no restrictions for use in the NHS per the drug's license, (2) no routine use (the drug is banned from NHS use altogether), or (3) restricted use only under certain circumstance, for certain patients, or in certain clinical indications narrower than the license. Of the 55 treatments appraised, 30 (55 percent) were approved without restrictions on their license, 16 (29 percent) were approved with restrictions, 8 (15 percent) were given no routine use, and one (2 percent) was not licensed (Mason and Drummond, 2008). Drugs that were restricted were most often approved for only a particular subset of patients. Alternatively, they were limited to use only in patients who responded while on them, as first- or second-line therapy only, or in patients who had not previously tried them. Reasons for these restrictions varied (Figure 6-5), and included insufficient evidence of effectiveness, methodological issues in economic analyses, uncertainty concerning the evidence submitted for the appraisal, an incremental cost-effectiveness ratio (ICER) that did not clearly meet NICE criteria, or an ICER that was too high.

Recent Controversy Surrounding NICE

NICE recently appraised several new drugs for treating renal carcinoma and recommended that none of them be used by the NHS because of poor cost-effectiveness.[2] There was uproar as a result, with oncologists and patients outraged that the drugs were not offered in the United Kingdom but were readily available in other countries. While there was speculation that NICE had become overly stringent in its decisions, Dr. Drummond

---

[2] Versus interferon alpha, one drug (sunitinib) cost £71,462 per QALY (£31,185 for 0.44 QALYs gained), a second (bevacizumab) cost £171,301 per QALY (£45,435 for 0.27 QALYs gained), and a third (temsirolimus) cost £94,385 per QALY (£22,272 for 0.24 QALYs gained) (NICE, 2008).

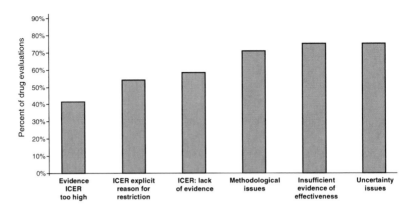

FIGURE 6-5 Reasons for NICE restrictions by percent of drug evaluations, May 2000 through March 2008 (n = 24).
SOURCES: Drummond presentation, February 9, 2009; Mason and Drummond, 2008.

explained that NICE had not changed its criteria at all. Instead, the cost of drugs submitted for appraisal had increased, and a greater number exceeded the cost-effectiveness threshold (Mason and Drummond, 2008).

These controversies surrounding NICE pose important questions:

1. How did NICE arrive at the threshold, and is the threshold at the correct cost-effectiveness level?
2. Are oncology drugs special in some way that should exempt them from NICE rules?

Regarding the first question, Dr. Drummond explained that the threshold is not based on research. Analysis of current cancer care expenditures in the NHS has found that the health service spends about £13,000 for every QALY gained—much less than the threshold (Martin et al., 2007). Ongoing research in the United Kingdom population is examining what the public thinks a QALY is worth and whether it is worth the same amount in different circumstances.

Regarding whether cancer drugs should be exempt from NICE rules, there has been a major development. Treatments can now qualify for what is called "supplementary guidance for end-of-life therapies" only if they are indicated for a small patient population with a life expectancy less than 24 months, if no equivalent active therapy exists, and if they would add at least three months to patients' life expectancy. For drugs recommended for approval in this manner, the QALYs gained assume full quality of life in the added months. Also, NICE's Appraisal Committee can take the view that, when adjusted this way, the QALYs gained at the end of life as a result of the treatment should be weighted highly enough for the therapy to be considered cost-effective when judged against the institute's existing cost-effectiveness threshold for approval. This compromise is based on the understanding that QALYs are worth more to those who have less time to live, or those who are very unfortunate health-wise. The application of this new guidance has led to approval of the drugs for renal cancer that were initially declined, although there were also additional negotiations between NICE and the manufacturers that contributed to this change.

Another approach has been the establishment of performance-related contracts, such as that for Velcade (bortezomib). During Velcade's technology appraisal, which appeared not to be going as well as hoped, the manufacturer approached NICE and offered to provide credit to the NHS for those patients who did not show a clinical response to the drug. Other manufacturers have done the same to try to reduce concerns among payors.

Dr. Drummond concluded that there is considerable variation across Europe both in access to drugs and the extent to which they are assessed for value. However, assessments like those performed by NICE are widely used in drug formulary listings and the assessments do lead to restrictions in the use of medications. There are two key issues: what is considered good value for the money, and whether cancer should be treated differently from other diseases.

DISCUSSION

Dr. Bhadrasain Vikram of the National Cancer Institute asked Dr. Newcomer why, with the huge data he had available to him at United-Healthcare, he did not simply perform his own NICE-like scientific approval designation. Dr. Newcomer explained that the insurance regulations in the United States vary from state to state, and this introduces many barriers to implementing uniform coverage decisions. He had found it very difficult to mandate that UnitedHealthcare not cover a drug because of expense or equivocal evidence.

Dr. John Mendelsohn of the M.D. Anderson Cancer Center asked whether NICE's guidance was only for the NHS or whether it also applied to the United Kingdom's private sector as well. Dr. Drummond explained that it applied almost entirely to the NHS because few of the technologies NICE has examined impact the largest applications of private health insurance in the United Kingdom, such as outpatient surgery, and few private payors followed the NHS' coverage decisions in the same way private payors in the United States follow decisions of the Centers for Medicare and Medicaid Services (CMS).

Dr. Robert Mass of Genentech asked how NICE integrates the value of innovation into its equation when assessing novel drugs. Dr. Drummond said that it was clearly in the guidance for the NICE committee to consider innovation in the drugs they assess, but many decisions revolve around the cost-effectiveness threshold. The French system, he said, has gone further toward pricing drugs based on their level of innovation. Dr. Neumann added that Medicare's national coverage decisions seem to be moving in the direction of considering innovation but hinge centrally on clinical outcomes. He noted that a treatment can be very innovative without necessarily being good value.

Dr. Tunis recalled while at CMS that he had seen data to suggest oncologists prescribe chemotherapy to increase personal income. He asked Dr. Neumann whether a self-report survey such as his could actually provide insights into personal revenue-driven prescribing. Dr. Neumann said that he and his colleagues tried to address this issue a number of ways, asking such questions in the survey as "To what extent have Medicare rules on oral chemotherapy limited your prescribing?" Around 60 percent said the Medicare rules had limited their prescribing. Dr. Neumann said the survey also asked oncologists whether they thought physicians in their profession made too much money. Few thought so. Dr. Neumann reported that he and his colleagues had also tried to identify the subset of respondents in practice settings with greater opportunity to make money by prescribing. Unfortunately, this was hard to tease out. Dr. Newcomer recalled an article in *Health Affairs* that suggested oncologists were not prescribing just to make money when there was not a reasonable indication, though they were maximizing revenue by choosing the more expensive regimen when they had multiple options (Jacobson et al., 2006).

Dr. Sargent was careful to note that Dr. Newcomer's standardization of practices was not a true cluster randomization design because there was no embedded randomization step. Dr. Sargent suggested that Dr. Newcomer introduce some element of randomization to the process and encouraged him to do some type of matching so that the study groups could be compared in valid ways. Dr. Newcomer agreed with these points. His first priority, though, was to encourage standardization of treatments because this alone could dramatically improve outcomes.

Dr. Mendelsohn pointed out that it should be the patient who decides the therapies she or he will receive. The physician is ethically required to present a balanced recommendation for therapy, but the physician cannot make the ultimate decision. Dr. Neumann agreed and added that more research was needed on how people think about small probabilities of large gains and how this influences their decisions.

REFERENCES

CEVR (Center for the Evaluation of Value and Risk in Health). 2009. *Cost-effectiveness analysis registry.* www.cearegistry.org (accessed April 11, 2009).

GAO (United States General Accounting Office). 1975. *Information on 1976 health insurance premium rate increases for federal employees health benefits program.* Washington, DC: United States Office of Personnel Management.

Jacobson, M., J. A. O'Malley, C. C. Earle, J. Pakes, P. Gaccione, and J. P. Newhouse. 2006. Does reimbursement influence chemotherapy treatment for cancer patients? *Health Affairs* 25(2):437–443.

Jonsson, B., and N. Wilking. 2007. Market uptake of new oncology drugs. *Annals of Oncology* 18(Suppl 3):18.

Martin, S., N. Rice, and P. C. Smith. 2007. *The link between health care spending and health outcomes: Evidence from English programme budgeting data. Research paper 24.* York, United Kingdom: Centre for Health Economics, University of York.

Mason, A. R., and M. Drummond. 2009. Public fundng of new cancer drugs: Is NICE getting nastier? *European Journal of Cancer* 45(7):1188–1192.

Nadler, E., B. Eckert, and P. J. Neumann. 2006. Do oncologists believe new cancer drugs offer good value? *The Oncologist* 11(2):90–95.

NICE (National Institute for Health and Clinical Excellence). 2008. *Renal cell carcinoma— Bevacizumab, sorafenib, sunitinib, and temsirolimus.* http://guidance.nice.org.uk/TA/Wave14/22 (accessed February 9, 2009).

Pusztai, L., and F. J. Esteva. 2006. Continued use of trastuzumab (Herceptin) after progression on prior trastuzumab therapy in HER-2-positive metastatic breast cancer. *Cancer Investigation* 24(2):187–191.

Reddy, J. C., J. D. Reimann, S. M. Anderson, and P. M. Klein. 2006. Concordance between central and local laboratory HER2 testing from a community-based clinical study. *Clinical Breast Cancer* 7(2):153–157.

Wennberg, J. E., E. S. Fisher, T. A. Stukel, J. S. Skinner, S. M. Sharp, and K. K. Bronner. 2004. Use of hospitals, physician visits, and hospice care during last six months of life among cohorts loyal to highly respected hospitals in the United States. *BMJ* 328(7440):607.

7

Ethical Issues and Value in Oncology

ETHICAL ISSUES WHEN CONSIDERING INSURANCE COVERAGE BASED ON VALUE IN THE TREATMENT OF CANCER

Dr. Daniel Brock of Harvard Medical School's Division of Medical Ethics began with his description of value in cancer care and treatment: "That the benefits in life extension and improved quality of life are obtained at a reasonable cost comparable to other typically-funded treatments and at a reasonable cost per quality-adjusted life-year (QALY)." Many cancer drugs fail to meet this standard, which is in essence a cost-effectiveness standard, he said.

How should resources be distributed to different health care needs and patients? The value answer to that question is based on cost-effectiveness, meaning that health care resources should be allocated to maximize health benefits from available resources to the population served, Dr. Brock explained. One way to approach cost-effectiveness is to limit the cost allowed for a unit of benefit. While the National Institute of Health and Clinical Excellence (NICE) in Britain uses a particular threshold, the United States spends about twice as much per capita on health care as what the United Kingdom spends, so there is no reason to use Britain's threshold. Roughly $100,000 per QALY is a threshold that many economists often apply, and it fits with the $6,000,000 to $7,000,000 for the value of a statistical life often used in health and safety regulations. Such a cost per

QALY cap represents one way to determine how to distribute health care resources, but many new cancer drugs cost two to three times this threshold of $100,000 per QALY.

Causes of Poor Cost-Effectiveness and Value Among Cancer Treatments

What are the causes of poor cost-effectiveness and value in cancer treatments? There are multiple causes, Dr. Brock said. First, the intellectual property protections and monopoly pricing afforded by 20 years of patent protection enables pharmaceutical manufacturers to set any price they want or believe they can get for a new drug. Second, though Medicare is the biggest purchaser of cancer drugs in this country, it is explicitly prohibited under part B from negotiating prices with drug companies. As a result of this prohibition, pharmaceutical manufacturers know that they will not be denied coverage by Medicare on grounds of cost. Most private insurance companies tend to follow Medicare's coverage decisions, meaning that they do not apply any cost-effectiveness standard either. Therefore, manufacturers have no incentive to develop cost-effective drugs and no incentive to price drugs in a cost-effective manner. Third, most cancer patients have health insurance, meaning that they tend to be concerned only with their out-of-pocket costs. With out-of-pocket costs making up just a fraction of the total cost to the health care system of an insured patient's care, there is little incentive for patients to reject care that is not cost-effective. Finally, some oncologists receive substantial income from using these new drugs for patients, and many physicians feel an obligation to do what is best for the patient no matter what the cost. All in all, said Dr. Brock, treatment decision makers (physicians and patients) have little incentive to weigh the true costs of care against the benefits, payors are largely precluded from negotiating for lower costs, and manufacturers have monopoly pricing to charge as much as they can get.

Regarding monopoly pricing, the usual justification has been that it is necessary so manufacturers will invest in research and development. This is a sound justification, said Dr. Brock. For some new cancer drugs, however, a different justification has been offered—that the prices reflect the value of the benefits of these drugs. In the setting of monopoly pricing, it is important that cost-per-QALY standards are caps rather than a price justified in this way. By analogy, suppose you were drowning and someone were on a dock ready to throw you a life ring. Can that person charge you a hundred thousand dollars or more for the life ring? Ethically speaking, the answer is clearly "no," said Dr. Brock. To do so would be to exploit someone's desperate circumstances. Therefore, the value benefit does not determine what price a service should have when one is not in a competitive market.

Ethical Justifications for Spending That Is Not Cost-Effective

After discussing these reasons for the failure of cost-effectiveness and value in cancer treatments, Dr. Brock moved to discuss ethical justifications for spending beyond what a cost-effectiveness threshold would dictate.

Adhering to the adage that one can tell the justice of a society by how it treats its least well-off members, special concern or priority is often given to those who are worst off. Does this justify spending more on cancer patients who are near death? In other words, are those with the worst health (those nearest death) truly those in the most urgent need? Dr. Brock explained that he thought these were not the patients who were the most in need based on equity considerations. Assume for a moment, Dr. Brock said, that giving cancer drugs is equivalent to providing additional months or years of life. Who are the worst off with respect to months and years of life? They are those who will have had the least life if they are not treated—this is not the elderly cancer patient but the younger patients. Consider 65-year-old patient A who will die in 1 month without a liver transplant and 35-year-old patient B who will die in 4 months without a liver transplant. Patient A is clearly more urgently ill, like the elderly advanced cancer patient, but patient B is worse off in the relevant sense because patient B will have had many fewer years of life if he or she doesn't get the transplant. Therefore, the most urgent are not the worst off, said Dr. Brock, and therefore urgent, dying cancer patients do not deserve special priority for medical interventions.

Dr. Brock asked how would one want to allocate the money for their health care over the course of a lifetime? One would not want to ask that question with only 3 months to live because that would bias the answer. From an unbiased point in their lives, it is probably not the case that people would want to allocate as much as $300,000 per QALY at the end of life. Put another way, should there be a special priority given to life extension over other health needs? The so-called rule of rescue coined by Al Jonsen (Jonsen, 1986) is often applied here. It states that we are unwilling to let an identified person in peril die or suffer great harm when we could rescue that person, even if it may be very costly. In an advanced cancer case, however, many expensive new drugs do not really rescue dying patients but only provide a small chance of life extension. This is not the type of benefit that the rule of rescue involves.

Another factor that influences resource allocation is the difference in how people think about real versus statistical lives. When saving statistical lives, by improving cancer screening for instance, one does not know and will likely never know whose lives will be saved. There are many cases in which improving rates of cancer screening would save more QALYs than many expensive chemotherapeutic treatments, but the benefits due to cancer drugs receive more attention. While we may be more moved by lives we can identify, statistical lives that we cannot identify should still receive as much moral and ethical importance as real lives, Dr. Brock said. Similarly, one should not place less value on future health benefits compared to acute benefits just because they come in the future. Investing in screening rather than acute interventions may be less appealing because the benefits will not be apparent until years later, and they are discounted because they are not immediately apparent. Determining value by cost-effectiveness with standard discounting of health benefits in this way gives undue importance to acute cancer interventions at the expense of prevention, and it gives undue weight to expensive, last-chance treatments.

Briefly touching on coinsurance, Dr. Brock described new fourth-tier insurance policies that typically require co-pays of a percentage of the total cost, as opposed to a fixed cost. Often these co-pays are on the order of 20 percent, and for an advanced-stage cancer patient with a $100,000 annual cost that amounts to $20,000 per year. Many patients are not able to afford this. So, while it may discourage some low-value uses of health care, coinsurance does so unethically because it prevents those who cannot pay from receiving care but only discourages or inconveniences the same health care use among those who can.

What Is Needed to Improve Value?

Dr. Brock said, "The most fundamental thing that is needed is willingness to—I'll use the *R* word—ration even last-chance care at the end of life. What is needed is a willingness not to cover very cost-marginal interventions, in particular at the end of life." It may not come easily or soon, and it will require major cultural changes in the thinking of those in health care, as well as the establishment of a national health care system to avoid the current variations in care.

In conclusion, Dr. Brock suggested smaller steps to improve value in cancer care. First, covering last-chance therapies only in clinical trials or for registry patients would provide us with more evidence of effectiveness. Authorizing CMS to negotiate drug prices would help reduce costs. Finally, transforming the comparative effectiveness program under consideration in Congress into a cost-effectiveness program would be a much larger step in the right direction.

CLINICIAN–PATIENT COMMUNICATION ABOUT CANCER THERAPY: ETHICAL ISSUES

Dr. Neil Wenger of the University of California at Los Angeles described his understanding of value in cancer care as "the net benefit of the treatment in terms of the goals of the patient, accounting for the negative effects of the treatment across all patients and considering the cost of the treatment. This includes the value of having a treatment, the opportunity costs of forgoing other treatments or of closure, and potential alternative uses of health care resources." This description of value focuses on the outcomes for the resources invested, is predicated on conserving and preserving resources for other valued activities, and incorporates elements of fairness, Dr. Wenger explained.

Moving on from this description of value, Dr. Wenger turned to an exploration of the clinical, ethical realities and challenges that affect value. He began with a clinical case (Box 7-1).

To operationalize value in cancer care means selecting to use some treatments and not using others. This requires transparency, an appeal mechanism, and enforcement, Dr. Wenger said (Daniels and Sabin, 2002).

It is also important to recognize that in order to compute the value in cancer care, we are generally dependent on outcome data from clinical trials. To the degree that cancer treatments are used outside of conditions established in their randomized controlled trials (RCTs), the cost-effectiveness data generated by the RCTs do not apply. There is a tremendous pressure to rescue in clinical cancer care, as evident in the case (Box 7-1) and "innovative" or off-label use of chemotherapeutic agents is common. While the RCT of erlotinib clearly showed a 2-month survival benefit and a 9 percent response rate for stage IIIB/IV non-small cell lung cancer (NSCLC) patients compared to less than 1 percent in the control arm (Shepherd et

BOX 7-1
A Clinical Case

A 55-year-old woman is transferred to the intensive care unit (ICU) after complications following resection of brain metastasis from her non-small cell lung cancer. She is a lawyer. She married late in life and has a young daughter. She never smoked. The patient and her husband traveled 40 miles, bypassing numerous other large hospitals with cancer programs, to receive cancer care at a particular academic center.

Twenty months ago, the patient was diagnosed with unresectable non-small cell lung cancer. She responded to six cycles of combination chemotherapy and then received maintenance bevacizumab treatment. One year after presentation, a full-body PET (positron emission tomography) scan showed no tumor activity.

Eighteen months after diagnosis, the patient was admitted to the hospital with altered mental status; an MRI scan at that time showed two frontal brain metastases. She underwent surgical resection of the brain metastases on hospital day 11 with post-op MRI imaging showing evidence of residual tumor.

The patient had a complicated post-operative course including intracerebral bleeding, a low blood platelet count, and deteriorating mental status on day 16 in the hospital. The ICU team was concerned that the aggressiveness of her care might be inappropriate. On hospital days 28 and 32, she underwent neurosurgical procedures to drain cerebral fluid collections associated with the tumor. On hospital day 47, the patient's respiratory function worsened due to pulmonary infection and the ICU team was concerned that she would require mechanical ventilation.

The primary oncologist discussed the patient's dire prognosis with the patient's husband, and he requested any available treatment. The primary oncologist explained that administration of erlotinib was an option, but he did not recommend this treatment, citing evidence that it provides only a 10 percent chance of response with an average 2-month life extension. The patient's husband requested continued ICU care so that his wife might receive—and perhaps benefit from—erlotinib treatment. On hospital day 53, imaging showed further intracerebral tumor progression. On hospital day 58, the patient's condition was stable enough to begin erlotinib treatment by nasogastric tube. On hospital day 62, she had worsening clinical status, hypertension, and renal failure. The relationship between the patient's husband and the ICU team became increasingly strained.

Discussions between the patient's husband and the primary oncologist then turned to comfort care, and on hospital day 64 the care goal was changed to palliation. The patient was moved out of the ICU and died comfortably the following day.

SOURCE: Wenger presentation, February 10, 2009.

al., 2005), this patient did not fit the inclusion criteria for this trial.[1] The patient's performance status (Oken et al., 1982) was far too low, and she had symptomatic brain metastases. While one might say the oncologist got the data from the RCT right, these data should not have been applied to this patient in this clinical situation; the $37,000 cost of the mean benefit shown in the erlotinib RCT (Carlson et al., 2008) is a tiny fraction of the expense required to maintain this patient to receive the medication.

Physicians have a powerful motivation to rescue. Dr. Wenger quoted Al Jonsen (Jonsen, 1986) saying, "Our moral response to the eminence of death demands that we rescue the doomed," and then added, "This rescue morality spills into medical care where our ropes are artificial hearts. Should the rule of rescue set a limit to rational calculation of the efficacy of technology?" Cancer patients are willing to pay the price—although they rarely pay all or even most of it—to achieve a personal rescue. Seriously ill patients with metastatic cancer are willing to accept a far greater burden for a small chance of benefit. In one study cancer patients were willing to withstand substantial side effects and risks for a 1 percent chance of cure, while physicians required a higher probability of benefit (10 percent), and nurses and the general public required a higher probability still (50 percent) (Agrawal and Emanuel, 2003). This tremendous demand for rescue at the end of life sets off a cascade of aggressive care, often without a discussion of prognosis or next steps for care or palliation in the event of clinical decline. When this decline arrives, the health care system meets it with intensive care, organ support, and, not infrequently, undignified suffering prior to the patient's death, which leads to pathological bereavement, poor health care practitioner morale, and high costs.

The virtue of a public decision-making mechanism to guide care in rescue situations would be its impartiality and balance of interests. Our individual intuition that we should rescue may not be the correct response from the societal perspective, Dr. Wenger said. Additionally, there is not a clear right that people have to be rescued. A question posed by Dr. Ramsey, Dr. Wenger said, is how willing are we to restrict access to marginally

---

[1] The erlotinib clinical trial inclusion criteria required patients 18 years or older; pathologic evidence of NSCLC; prior combination chemotherapy; the absence of other malignancies, cardiac disease, and gastrointestinal or ophthalmologic abnormalities; the absence of symptomatic brain metastases; and an Eastern Cooperative Oncology Group (ECOG) performance status measure between 1 and 3, meaning included patients would at least be capable of performing some self-care.

beneficial cancer therapies because they are too costly for what they do (Ramsey, 2007)? Dr. Wenger reframed the question to ask: To whom does this responsibility fall—insurance carriers? Physicians?

In a statement endorsed by multiple professional medical associations entitled *Medical Professionalism in the New Millennium: A Physician Charter* (*Charter*), the fundamental element of a physician's professional responsibility is the principle of primacy of patient welfare. This principle is founded on dedication to serving the interests of the patient and an altruism that builds trust, which is central to the physician–patient relationship (ABIM Foundation et al., 2002). Market forces, societal pressures, and administrative exigencies are not to compromise this principle, Dr. Wenger read from the *Charter*. Following this principle of the primacy of patient welfare, the very next principle is the principle of social justice, Dr. Wenger said, which requires that physicians promote the fair distribution of finite clinical resources and provide health care based on wise, cost-effective management while meeting the needs of individual patients. The *Charter* continues, "The provision of unnecessary services not only exposes one's patients to avoidable harm and expense, but also diminishes the resources available for others" (ABIM Foundation et al., 2002). So, this *Charter* indicates that at least some of the responsibility to limit costly, ineffective treatment falls to clinicians.

Numerous studies both in the United States and internationally have shown that patients sometimes want cancer treatment that clinicians might not be willing to accept for themselves due to high toxicities and low probability of benefit at the end of life (Matsuyama et al., 2006). Furthermore, while a patient's prognostic estimate and their desire for aggressive, life-sustaining treatment both decrease as the end of life nears, patients' prognostic estimates are often unrealistically optimistic (Weeks et al., 1998). What responsibility do clinicians bear for these optimistic patient prognostic estimates? Many factors play a role: (1) oncologists tend to be optimists themselves, (2) prognostication is difficult, and (3) empathic discussions of prognosis, adverse health outcomes, and costs are difficult. Such discussions of prognosis infrequently happen in a timely manner, even though the evidence suggests that patients want this information and guidance in cancer care decisions.

Physicians are able to provide the guidance patients want in cancer care decisions, Dr. Wenger said. An article coauthored by Tom Smith (Harrington and Smith, 2008), Dr. Wenger recalled, describes ways to help orient patients toward care at the end of life and outlines the questions that physicians might have patients ask them in order to elicit all the information that might be needed to guide care and use resources appropriately (Table 7-1).

Gruen and colleagues have presented the ways that socioeconomic factors influence individual patients' health and their relation to the physician's core professional responsibility for patient care (Gruen et al., 2004; Figure 7-1). They posit that the physician's responsibilities go beyond shepherding individual patient care, extending to obligations to ensure access

TABLE 7-1 Helpful Questions for Patients with Advanced Cancer to Consider Asking Their Oncologists

Questions About Treatment	Questions About Prognosis
What is my chance of cure?	What are the likely things that will happen to me?
What is the chance that this chemotherapy will make my cancer shrink? Stay stable? Grow?	How long will I live? (ask for a range and the most likely scenario for the period ahead)
If I cannot be cured, will I live longer with chemotherapy? How much longer?	Are there things I should be doing? Making a will? Making an advance directive? Deciding upon a durable power of attorney for health care who can speak for me, if I am unable? Addressing financial or family legal issues? Appointing a durable power of attorney for financial affairs? Establishing a trust?
What are the main side effects of the chemotherapy?	
Will I feel better or worse?	
Are there other options, such as hospice or palliative care?	
How do other people make these decisions?	
Are there clinical trials available? What are the benefits? Am I eligible? What is needed to enroll?	Family issues Will you help me talk with my children?
	Spiritual and psychological issues Who is available to help me cope with this situation?
	Legacy and life review What do I want to pass on to my family to tell them about my life?
	Other concerns?

SOURCES: Wenger presentation, February 10, 2009; Harrington and Smith, 2008.

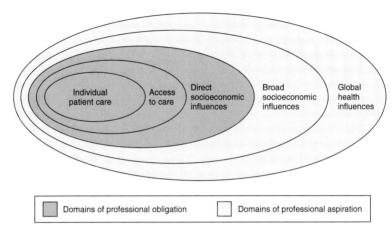

FIGURE 7-1 Model of physician responsibility in relation to influences on health.
SOURCES: Wenger presentation, February 10, 2009; Gruen et al., 2004.

to care and to effect socioeconomic forces with direct influence on health
(shaded inner ovals, Figure 7-1). According to this model, the oncologist's
stewardship role at the community level should be to participate in decisions regarding the appropriate use of cancer resources, to work with health
care teams in deciding reasonable options while maintaining a continuity
role, to participate in setting limits, to participate in quality improvement
efforts, and to aid in policy decisions regarding appropriate care within one's
catchment area, Dr. Wenger said. Dr. Wenger then returned to the patient
discussed in his presentation, a 55-year-old woman with brain metastases
who received erlotinib in the ICU with little chance of benefit. What was
really needed, Dr. Wenger said, was the presence of an oncologist who
would fill those roles—guiding care, setting limits, and participating in
quality improvement efforts.

Dr. Wenger recalled a discussion with the patient's husband (Box 7-1)
after the patient's death. He said,

> I needed to hear from our oncologist that the treatment should stop, that it
> would not help; not that there was something that we could do or might do.
> Although I desperately wanted my wife to survive, she and I would even have
> selected not to have the brain surgery if it was unlikely to help. They needed
> to say, "You're dying. This is what you should do." My daughter never got to
> be with her mommy in the end. I still don't know what to say to her.

In conclusion, Dr. Wenger said, the physician's role in guiding cancer care is far broader than selecting the right chemotherapeutic agents—it is to inform patients and surrogates about the course, risks, and benefits of treatment in an iterative, ongoing fashion. It is to discuss prognosis, if the patient is willing, and to provide continuity of guidance. It is to work with care teams in deciding reasonable treatment options, and to participate in deciding appropriate use of cancer care resources on the policy level. This includes guiding patients to receive care that best meets their goals within the constraints of policy-level decisions, discussing cost, and disclosing potential conflicts of interest.

What if, Dr. Wenger asked, oncology's role in guiding and providing care Americans need was to delineate fair and appropriate costs for cancer care resources at the policy level? What if oncologists took the lead on a social exploration of when resource-based rules might be suspended for rescue? What if oncologists as a group demanded that the structure of routine care yield data to improve treatment and explain the shortcomings of current standard approaches?

DISCUSSION

Dr. Patricia Ganz of the University of California, Los Angeles, compared the pressure to prescribe aggressive chemotherapy to the pressure to prescribe antibiotics for viral illnesses. In both situations, the clinician feels that it is simpler to provide a prescription than to leave patients with none. She mentioned an innovative solution pediatricians have developed to address the pressure they felt to prescribe antibiotics: prescription pads for supportive care therapeutic interventions to treat viral illnesses. By analogy, oncology societies including American Society of Clinical Oncology (ASCO) should play an important role in making sure that palliative care can be made available in a similar way as an alternative prescription to give patients, instead of chemotherapy with little chance for benefit. The hospice benefit should also be made available to patients starting their first course of chemotherapy for advance-stage malignancies so that oncologists are not forced to say "I have nothing else to give or do for you" before handing the patient off to another team.

Dr. Ferrell emphasized the difficulties faced by those who lacked health insurance or had gone bankrupt due to large co-pays. Dr. Ferrell recalled the story of a colleague who had been an oncology nurse for 30 years prior to being diagnosed with her third primary cancer when she lost her job and insurance because of her illness. She had lost nearly everything she owned, and the cost of her chemotherapy was over $10,000 per month. During an outpatient visit to receive her chemotherapy, Dr. Ferrell said, the colleague got up out of bed, had an episode of syncope, and collapsed. Staff in the clinic called a code, anticipating the need to resuscitate her, and one staff member began to wheel the crash cart toward the collapsed woman. On the floor, the colleague woke up and saw the clinic team running toward her with the crash cart. When she realized what was going on, she immediately began to try desperately to prevent the clinic team from opening the crash cart, mouthing the words as clearly as she could while still nearly incapacitated on the ground. She did this because she knew that breaking the seal on the crash cart would cost her another $1,000 out-of-pocket. This awful scenario is what our system has produced today, Dr. Ferrell concluded.

Dr. Rossi said that he thought everyone at the workshop could agree that trying to assess value and determine whether we are getting value for the money is critical for the health care system. He asked the speakers whether there was an ethical requirement upon pharmaceutical companies to enter markets where there are differential standards of care purely to gain access to markets where a product is already being used off label. Dr. Brock thought that clinical trials of pharmaceuticals ought to benefit the community they are performed in, but it is ethically problematic for companies to put themselves in positions where the only way they can satisfy the study populations is to have a successful outcome and validate the existing off-label use of a drug.

Dr. Max Coppes of the Children's National Medical Center asked whether legal constraints and the pressure to practice defensive medicine force oncologists to make decisions that lead to low value. Dr. Wenger said there was no doubt this was the case. There is constantly a tension between doing the right thing and doing the defensive thing in clinical practice. That is why there is a need for standards of care established by the profession. Dr. Brock added that the problem of defensive medicine is not driven just by concerns over malpractice, but it is reinforced by a medical culture that teaches trainees to run unnecessary tests and drive diagnostic uncertainty as close to zero as possible.

Ms. Alison Smith of C-Change asked whether advance directives could be used as a vehicle to proactively assess a patient's vision of value. Dr. Wenger replied that advance directives are tools to help in guiding care and should be used by oncologists. Dr. Brock cited the SUPPORT trial (SUPPORT Principal Investigators, 1995), adding that completing an advance directive is not enough. In addition, physicians need to have more discussions about the end of life with their patients, and they need to adhere to the advance directives once they are written.

REFERENCES

ABIM Foundation, ACP–ASIM Foundation, and European Federation of Internal Medicine. 2002. Medical professionalism in the new millennium: A physician charter. *Annals of Internal Medicine* 136(3):243–246.

Agrawal, M., and E. J. Emanuel. 2003. Ethics of phase I oncology studies: Reexamining the arguments and data. *Journal of the American Medical Association* 290(8):1075–1082.

Carlson, J. J., C. Reyes, N. Oestreicher, D. Lubeck, S. D. Ramsey, and D. L. Weenstra. 2008. Comparative clinical and economic outcomes of treatments for refractory non-small-cell lung cancer (NSCLC). *Lung Cancer* 61(3):405–415.

Daniels, N., and J. E. Sabin. 2002. *Setting limits fairly: Can we learn to share medical resources?* New York: Oxford University Press.

Gruen, R. L., S. D. Pearson, and T. A. Brennan. 2004. Physician-citizens—Public roles and professional obligations. *Journal of the American Medical Association* 291(1):94–98.

Harrington, S. E., and T. J. Smith. 2008 The role of chemotherapy at the end of life: "When is enough, enough?" *Journal of the American Medical Association* 299(22):2667–2678.

Jonsen, A. R. 1986. Bentham in a box: Technology assessment and health care allocation. *Law, Medicine, and Health Care* 14(3–4):172–174.

Matsuyama, R., S. Reddy, and T. J. Smith. 2006. Why do patients choose chemotherapy near the end of life? A review of the perspective of those facing death from cancer. *Journal of Clinical Oncology* 24(21):3490–3496.

Oken, M. M., R. H. Creech, D. C. Tormey, J. Horton, T. E. Davis, E. T. McFadden, and P. P. Carbone. 1982. Toxicity and response criteria of the Eastern Cooperative Group. *American Journal of Clinical Oncology* 5(6):649–655.

Ramsey, S. D. 2007. How should we pay the piper when he's calling the tune? On the long-term affordability of cancer care in the United States. *Journal of Clinical Oncology* 25(2):175–179.

Shepherd, F. A., J. R. Pereira, T. Ciulenu, E. H. Tan, V. Hirsh, S. Thongprasert, D. Campos, S. Maoleekoonpiroj, M. Smylie, R. Martins, M. van Kooten, M. Dediu, B. Findlay, D. Tu, D. Johnston, A. Bezjak, G. Clark, P. Santabarbara, L. Seymour, and National Cancer Institute of Canada Clinical Trials Group. 2005. Erlotinib in previously treated non-small-cell lung cancer. *New England Journal of Medicine* 353(2):123–132.

SUPPORT Principal Investigators. 1995. A controlled trial to improve care for seriously ill hospitalized patients. The Study to Understand Prognoses and Preferences for Outcomes and Risks of Treatments (SUPPORT). *Journal of the American Medical Association* 274(20):1591–1598.

Weeks, J. C., E. F. Cook, S. J. O'Day, L. M. Peterson, N. Wenger, D. Reding, F. E. Harrell, P. Kussin, N. V. Dawson, A. F. Connors, J. Lynn, and S. R. Phillips. 1998. Relationship between cancer patients' predications of prognosis and their treatment preferences. *Journal of the American Medical Association* 279(21):1709–1714.

PART II:

SOLUTIONS FOR VALUE IN CANCER CARE

8

Improving Value in Oncology Practice: Ways Forward

VALUE-BASED INSURANCE DESIGN: INITIATIVES OUTSIDE OF ONCOLOGY

Dr. Michael Chernew of Harvard Medical School described value as a reflection of both cost and quality, making clear that value is not synonymous with either high quality or low cost alone. Measures of value and value-based initiatives must consider both jointly. Value-based insurance design (VBID) focuses on patient incentives and charges patients less for services that are of high value. The basic idea is simple: when we know a health care service is beneficial and of high value, we want to put as few financial barriers as possible between it and patients who it will benefit. By the same token, patients should bear a greater financial burden for care that has marginal value so as to encourage efficiency. VBID recognizes that patient demand and preferences should play a role in the care delivered and that patients should share some of the financial burden, but it also recognizes that standard economic demand theory should not be blindly applied. In this way, VBID is a hybrid of economics and incentive design, with the recognition that the health care market does not operate according to standard market rules. Also, it is important to distinguish VBID from value-based purchasing, which tends to focus on the way providers are paid and incentivized (Chernew et al., 2007, 2008; Fendrick et al., 2001).

Insurance Theory

Insurance lowers prices at the point of service and alleviates risk. The problem is that insured consumers buy services they would not otherwise buy if they were fully informed and had to pay the full price. This problem is termed *moral hazard*, and it drives people to consume excess care and leads to high premiums when patients are insulated from the full costs of care. Models of cost sharing should not be designed to lower premiums but rather to improve patient incentives and reduce excess use while encouraging price shopping. Optimal insurance would balance moral hazard's tendency for overuse and risk aversion, meaning that it would reduce co-pays in situations where the benefit of care justifies the expense and increase co-pays for care whose value does not justify the expense. This encourages patients to consume services that are high value and reduce use of inappropriate services. But patients do not respond to cost sharing as economists would like. Instead, greater cost sharing leads to patient reductions in the use of appropriate and inappropriate services alike, and this leads to worse outcomes (Siu et al., 1986).

Dr. Chernew reviewed VBID in areas of medicine other than cancer. An important dimension of a VBID program, he said, is the services it targets for lower co-pays, such as important medications for chronic illnesses. Pitney Bowes has become the model for targeting chronic illness services (Freudenheim, 2007; Fuhrmans, 2004). The University of Michigan has gone one step further to discount co-pays not just for important services such as diabetes medications but also for belonging to certain patient programs. A second important dimension of a VBID program is its scope: will the program simply lower co-pays for high-value services or also raise co-pays for low-value services? It is important to recognize that VBID tends to cost more money if co-pays are only lowered because it leads to greater use of services and a greater employer share of spending for high-value services that would be used whether or not VBID were in place. Advocates of VBID say that we can pay for VBID's extra spending because it leads to fewer adverse events and emergency department visits. The question is how many fewer adverse events will we have? VBID design will be more successful and the cost of VBID can be further offset if the patients targeted are at high risk for adverse events. The cost of VBID is further offset by benefits in patient productivity—important benefits that should not be overlooked. Another way to offset the costs of VBID is to increase the co-pays for low-value services or to implement a relatively small increase in cost over all services that are not deemed as having a high value. Dr. Chernew recalled a quote from David Meltzer that said, "If you are only doing VBID in situations where it saves money, you are not doing enough of it." We want to provide high-value care, and high-value care will not necessarily save money.

Results from the Literature on Value-Based Insurance Design

In a study of the impact of VBID on adherence to medications for chronic illnesses, co-pays for ACE inhibitors, beta-blockers, blood glucose control medications, statins, and inhaled corticosteroids were reduced significantly by a large employer. Co-pays for generic drugs were reduced to $0 from $5 and brand-name drug co-pays were reduced by half. As a result, adherence to all of the medications improved significantly (Figure 8-1).

After implementing VBID, Pitney Bowes claimed to save 6 percent in overall diabetes costs, or over $1 million total (Mahoney, 2005). A VBID program from Asheville, North Carolina, reduced annual diabetes costs per participant by $1,200 to $1,872 (Cranor et al., 2003). Another program for public employees in California increased co-pays and found that they were able to save 20 cents for every dollar spent on extra drugs; the program

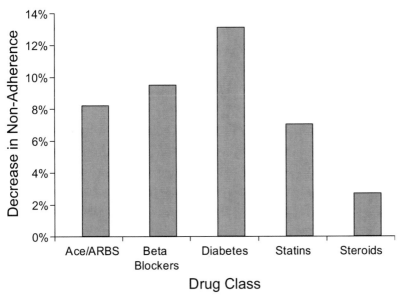

FIGURE 8-1 The impact of value-based insurance design upon adherence to ACE inhibitor, beta-blocker, glucose control, statin, and inhaled corticosteroid therapies. SOURCES: Chernew presentation, February 10, 2009; Chernew et al., 2008.

was also able to save up to 50 cents for every dollar among a subset of less healthy individuals (Chandra et al., 2007). In addition to increased use of high-value services, these studies show that cost savings to patients and employers are possible using VBID. Dr. Chernew said that he believed a well-designed VBID program could save money from a societal perspective as well, especially if it raised co-pays for low-value services. The productivity gains and savings from reduced disability would give even greater savings. Furthermore, better targeting through personalized medicine would have the potential to save money as well, especially in cancer care.

Applying Value-Based Insurance Design to Cancer

For VBID in cancer care, Dr. Chernew suggested that the first dollar co-pay be waived. Charging for the first dollar of services only serves to tax those unfortunate enough to be diagnosed with cancer. Instead, increase cost sharing on treatments that are of less value. Next, Dr. Chernew suggested that co-pays should be kept low for appropriate cancer screening services. In addition, if low-value care services can be identified, cancer patients should be charged more for those services. Finally, we can gain considerable value by pursuing personalized medicine, and there is great potential for personalizing cancer care.

Health care costs cannot grow at the rate they have grown historically. The question is how many people are going to be adversely affected when we slow health care spending growth? As a society we should make sure to slow health care growth in a way that minimizes adverse consequences and allows people access to high-value care. If we do not have the courage to determine what has high value and what does not, we will simply discourage use of services indiscriminately, and that would risk driving patients to lower-value care instead of promoting health care that is of high value.

GENERATING EVIDENCE OF VALUE POST-FDA APPROVAL: IS THERE A ROLE FOR HEALTH INSURERS?

Reducing Uncertainty to Improve Value

Dr. Tunis explained that his presentation would be focused on understanding uncertainty in clinical benefits, a topic infrequently discussed while considering value. Though value can be described in many different ways, every description rests on the existence of some measure of benefit to someone, whether through improved outcomes, hope, opportunity, or innovation. Furthermore, every measure of benefit has some degree of uncertainty about the magnitude of the benefit. How confident we are in what we know about the benefits of medical care directly affects how we talk about value, but too little consideration is given to our uncertainty. Whether in extrapolating overall survival from time-to-progression data or in determining the precise extent of clinical benefit for cost-effectiveness decisions, reducing this underlying uncertainty around clinical benefits can help us assess the value of care.

We also fail to get the best value from our health care system in part due to uncertainty, Dr. Tunis said, and we avoid discussing just how little we actually know about things that are important in care. Critical evidence gaps are common. In 2007, the number of randomized controlled trials (RCTs) published in the medical literature was 18,000. Despite all of this evidence being generated, the conclusion of every systematic review seems to be the same: the available evidence is limited by poor quality and further research is necessary. With 18,000 trials published every year and every review concluding that the evidence is limited, one begins to wonder how we could miss the target so often. How is this possible, and why does it happen? One would expect that we could find good evidence at least once in a while.

We all recognize that there are information gaps in health care that lead to uncertainty and problems improving value, but, Dr. Tunis joked, one cannot really explain anything these days without describing its molecular basis. Dr. Tunis then shared his discovery of the molecular basis of uncertainty (Figure 8-2).

Turning to Figure 8-2, Dr. Tunis explained that the uncertainty pathway begins with intellectual curiosity that feeds clinical research, which in turn produces published studies and information that slowly travel by passive diffusion (knowledge translation route 1 [KT1]) to reach policy decision makers inside the cell cytoplasm. Alternatively, health technology assessment can act as an active transport mechanism (knowledge translation route 2 [KT2]) to deliver information to (intracellular) policy makers. Because the evidence that reaches policy decision makers is often limited and imperfect, there are many gaps in the evidence, but a defective knowledge translation mechanism (KT3) prevents the information needs of decision makers from reaching the clinical research enterprise. As a result, we have a clinical research enterprise trying to push information into the cell but no feedback loop to transmit what decision makers really need to

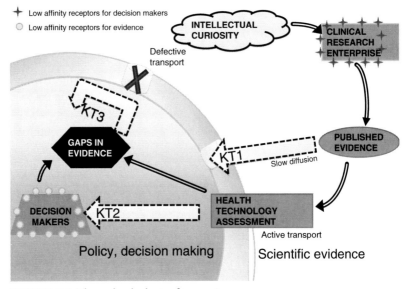

FIGURE 8-2 The molecular basis of uncertainty.
SOURCE: Tunis presentation, February 10, 2009.

know back out into the research enterprise. The communication difficulties are compounded by low-affinity receptors for evidence that surround policy makers and low-affinity receptors for policy makers that surround clinical research. Clearly, what we need is a targeted therapeutic to reduce uncertainty, Dr. Tunis said.

How do we create a better link between the evidence-generating enterprise and the policy makers who use that evidence to make the information delivered more responsive to existing needs or gaps? The Centers for Medicare and Medicaid Services (CMS) has a lengthy history of involvement in generating better evidence for policy decision making, from the investigational device exemption for coverage of certain devices in clinical trials (1996), to coverage for routine costs for patient care in clinical trials (2000), to ad hoc efforts to work with the National Institutes of Health (NIH). These efforts and many others reflect Medicare's transition from an agency that simply paid bills in the past to one with a much more important role of informing decision makers with evidence.

CMS's definition of what is clinically reasonable and necessary also drives research focused on policy decision making. For decades, Medicare had no standard definition for what it meant for a health care intervention to be clinically reasonable and necessary. In the year 2000, CMS began to define reasonable and necessary health care as that which has adequate evidence to conclude that the item or service improves net health outcomes. This was adopted on the basis of recurrent use, and it marked the first time that services CMS paid for would have to be supported by evidence that they improved outcomes. CMS then went further to say that the outcomes improved should be those that patients experience, such as quality of life, functional status, and so on. In effect, this explicit definition of reasonable and necessary health care also strongly influences how product developers and clinical researchers generate studies, pushing them toward reducing uncertainty around the issues that decision makers and patients actually care about.

Building Evidence for Health Care Technologies and Services After FDA Approval

The accretion of information and evidence for a technology or service occurs in a continuous fashion over time, Dr. Tunis said. From the time of its discovery, there is a certain amount that one knows about the technology by the time of its Food and Drug Administration (FDA) approval, and, it is hoped, more is known by the time it is covered by payors. But even then there remain many unanswered questions about the technology's long-term effects, risks, and other outcomes that will not be apparent until the technology becomes standard of care. The trouble is that further studies of a particular technology are discouraged once Medicare and commercial payors have made the decision to cover the technology. How then can we efficiently continue to learn about technologies and reduce uncertainty *after* insurers decide it should be paid for?

Coverage with evidence development (CED) is Medicare's attempt to reduce uncertainty by linking reimbursement for emerging, promising technologies to a requirement for prospective data collection on those technologies through clinical research studies. Medicare retains the authority to approve the design to those clinical studies based on whether they are sufficiently robust to allow Medicare to decide whether the technology is clinically reasonable and necessary and improves health outcomes for patients. For instance, CED was applied to off-label uses of drugs for colorectal cancer and stipulated that Medicare would only pay for the drugs if patients were enrolled in National Cancer Institute (NCI)-sponsored clinical trials. CED has also been applied to other emerging technologies, from FDG-PET (fluoro-D-glucose positron emission tomography) scans in oncology to implantable artificial hearts as an alternative to heart transplant. The results of CED have been modest, but there remains considerable policy interest in the CED concept.

Take for example CED for implantable cardiac defibrillators (ICDs), devices implanted in the chest wall to deliver an electrical impulse in the event of sudden cardiac arrest. While each ICD costs roughly $50,000, only about 20 percent of implanted ICDs ever need to fire. Coverage for ICDs was expanded in 2005 only for patients enrolled in a large national registry, and data submission to the registry was required for ICD reimbursement through Medicare. The number of patients in the registry has grown to 250,000–300,000, and there is hope that studying the registry data will help identify high-risk patients and predict the 20 percent of ICDs that will ultimately fire. In order to risk-stratify ICD patients in the future, the researchers will need baseline data (present in the registry) and follow-up data on which patients' ICDs fired. To date, the follow-up firing data has yet to be collected, chiefly because there is controversy about where this data should be stored. This is just one example of a hurdle that CED has faced.

CED has faced a number of other challenges. The first is timing—when coverage is under review, it may be too late to begin discussing CED. Second, it is difficult to design randomized studies for a treatment that is covered by insurance. Third, while payors see CED as an opportunity for coverage expansion for certain products, manufacturers see the opposite—a coverage limitation. Fourth, it is unclear how to fund the research CED promotes. Dr. Tunis emphasized the importance of removing CED considerations from the context of any specific coverage or payment decision and beginning the CED from early in the evolution of a technology. By the time the technology is considered more than just a promising new treatment modality, it is probably too late to restrict its use to clinical trials.

These challenges are not insurmountable, said Dr. Tunis, and there is work underway to build evidence for emerging technologies already on the market. Groups such as Dr. Tunis's Center for Medical Technology Policy (CMTP) and others are pursuing this work in areas where treatment methodologies have rarely been studied side by side, and significant gaps in clinical knowledge still exist, such as in the treatment of clinically localized prostate cancer (Wilt et al., 2008). The CMTP convened a variety of stakeholder groups around FDA-approved prostate cancer treatments and was preparing to study the various modalities head-to-head to gain better evidence of comparative effectiveness. Understanding value depends on reliable information, Dr. Tunis concluded. To get this reliable information and improve value, we are going to have to find better mechanisms for generating the information that policy makers are looking for.

COMMUNICATING EFFECTIVELY WITH CANCER PATIENTS ABOUT THE BENEFITS AND RISKS OF CANCER TREATMENTS

On the one hand, communicating with cancer patients about the risks, benefits, and costs might seem easy. Physicians can tell someone how an intervention might influence their survival and their quality of life and can present the risks, including financial costs, so that people should be able to decide how to weigh all of these risks and benefits to arrive at a decision. It seems straightforward, but clearly it is not, said Dr. Peter Ubel of the University of Michigan. Patient comprehension is not perfect, especially during discussions with significant emotional content, such as in cancer prognosis or end-of-life discussions. Furthermore, even with perfect comprehension of information, there may be other factors that influence how patients arrive at decisions.

Improving Comprehension

When conveying risks and benefits, clinicians should start by assessing a patient's comprehension. One major barrier to comprehension is innumeracy. For instance, if 10 percent of 1,000 people have a particular disease, only one in three Americans can calculate how many people actually have that condition (100 of the 1,000 people). Therefore, one should not assume that patients understand the concept of percentages. In fact, it may be better to assume the opposite.

When helping people make complicated decisions, information should be reinforced in multiple ways. Percentages should be reinforced with frequencies, and any numerical information should be reinforced visually. Pictographs improve comprehension better than other visual aids, such as bar graphs or pie charts, because pictographs help people quickly grasp the information relevant to their decision. For instance, the difference between outcomes of hormonal therapy with and without chemotherapy for breast cancer is more understandable when presented as a pictograph rather than a bar graph (Figure 8-3). In Figure 8-3 it is clear from the pictograph that adding chemotherapy translates into the survival of 2 more patients in every 100 even without the accompanying explanation. The pictograph presents the difference in risk, as opposed to a presenting the viewer with levels of

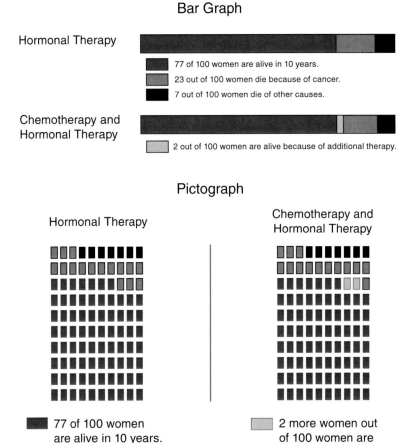

FIGURE 8-3 Statistical representation of the added mortality benefit of chemotherapy for breast cancer in addition to hormone therapy using a bar graph versus a pictograph; statistical benefit shown as 2 more women out of 100 alive because of additional chemotherapy.
SOURCE: Ubel presentation, February 9, 2009.

risk for each treatment which would then need to be compared. Performing this comparison for the viewer eliminates a computational step and improves comprehension and understanding.

Comprehension Is Not Enough

Comprehension is not always enough to ensure that the right decision is made. Even with perfect comprehension, a number of unconscious biases can lead people to decisions that do not follow from the information they have been provided. For instance, consider what happened when a group of women tried to decide whether to take tamoxifen for breast cancer prevention. Dr. Ubel and colleagues presented one group of such women with a pictograph showing the risk of developing cataracts as 11.3 out of 100. He presented a different group the same statistical information using different denominators (one showing the same cataract risk of 113 out of 1,000). These latter women were more worried about cataracts because they saw more boxes shaded in (113 compared to 11.3) even though the percentage had not changed. The pictograph with a denominator of 1,000 made the women "feel" as though the risk was greater, even though the risk was no different than the previous pictograph with a denominator of 100. So how can providers align what patients feel with the statistical information they must use to make decisions?

Human beings evolved without the written word and without numbers, explained Dr. Ubel. Instead, our ancestors told narrative stories to convey information, and this is how we are wired. Can stories or testimonials be used to improve comprehension of statistics? To illustrate the effect of stories on decisions involving statistical comprehension, Dr. Ubel described a study he had performed in which subjects were asked to imagine they had severe angina and were to decide between bypass surgery or angioplasty for treatment. Subjects were told that bypass would require open surgery, have a long recovery period, and a 75 percent chance of curing the angina, while angioplasty would require minimal surgery, a shorter recovery period, and a 50 percent chance of cure. In addition, subjects were provided two short testimonials for each treatment, one story of someone who was cured and one story of someone who was not for both bypass and angioplasty. Twenty percent of subjects chose bypass. Next, Dr. Ubel changed the experiment to reinforce the statistics with the testimonials. For bypass, subjects were provided with three stories of cure and one story in which the angina persisted (3 out of 4 or 75 percent) which reinforced the 75 percent success rate statistic subjects were given for bypass treatment. For angioplasty, two stories told of a cure and two did not, matching the 50 percent success rate given for the treatment. With the stories better aligned with the statistics, subjects chose bypass twice as often as before, or 41 percent of the time. When subjects were then given statistics *and* pictographs with or without testimonials to match the statistics, there was almost no difference in the number who chose bypass—38 percent and 44 percent chose bypass, respectively. Why was there no added benefit to adding testimonials once the pictographs were provided? Were both the testimonials and the pictographs effectively changing the way the statistical risks felt to subjects? Because the statistics were simple enough for high comprehension even without a pictograph and the choice of treatment was not associated with the level of numeracy of the subjects, Dr. Ubel concluded that, indeed, the pictographs helped subjects both comprehend and feel the difference in treatment success rates.

In conclusion, Dr. Ubel turned his attention to the social context of cancer care and clinical discussions of cost. He asked, is there a harder context to discuss costs than when faced with a life-threatening illness such as cancer? Comparing risks of mortality and quality of life can be challenging enough. Adding cost considerations seems almost inappropriate because most people have no way to conceptualize trade-offs between survival and cost. Physicians may have good methods available for communicating medical risks and benefits to patients, but the next big challenge is learning how to help patients factor in financial costs as well.

CONCRETE IDEAS FOR INCREASING VALUE
IN ONCOLOGY CARE: A VIEW FROM THE TRENCHES

Dr. Smith began by saying that his presentation would address a number of topics, including unrealistic demands for treatment benefit, low reimbursement for cognitive care, high reimbursement for chemotherapy or infusions, the high-income expectations of oncologists, variable quality, and stress and burnout.

Oncology Practice Problems, Their Explanations,
and How They Relate to Value

The United States spends twice as much money as any other country for the same results in treating cancer (Meropol and Schulman, 2007). While the system rewards oncologists for giving more and more treatment, rather than taking the time to explain to patients when more treatment will not help, the expectations for success in oncology are impossible to meet. As a result, 16–20 percent of patients receive chemotherapy within 14 days of death, hospice stays are too short (one third are only 3 days or less), and we spend 25 percent of Medicare dollars in the last months of life (Harrington and Smith, 2008). Meanwhile, there are at least 100 new cancer drugs in phase III clinical trials, all will be expensive—$5,000 to 7,000 per month (Hillner and Smith, 2009)—and many may be very useful. Allowing these same financial incentives to persist will not be sustainable, Dr. Smith said.

Unrealistic Demand for Benefit

Most people have unrealistic expectations of benefit from cancer care because they are told the goals of care but they are not told if they are going to die from the disease, how long they have to live, and the anticipated benefit from chemotherapy versus supportive care. The absence of decision aids for treatment of metastatic disease, or other tools to help clinicians weigh toxicities and cost when cure is not the goal, also enables unrealistic benefit expectations. As a result of this avoidant behavior, it is intellectually simpler and more financially rewarding to continue giving chemotherapy until the end is near obvious. By Dr. Smith's calculations, oncologists make three to five times more money by giving chemotherapy than by talking with people.

Low Reimbursement for Cognitive Care

Oncologists are paid based on relative value units (RVUs). At $37 per work-related RVU, an oncologist would have to generate over 16,000 work-related RVUs yearly to earn the average U.S. oncologist's salary. Most oncologists can do between 6,000 and 9,000 RVUs. Even if an oncologist could generate that many work-related RVUs, that would only cover his or her individual salary. How would the rest of the practice be supported? Other clinicians (nurses, social workers, counselors) and integral services (billing, electronic medical records, capital expenses, and so on) would not be supportable financially. Realistic workloads for long clinic days would lead to a decrease of roughly $200,000 per year in the average oncologist's income if they were based solely on cognitive services, and there would be no way to pay oncologists' staff.

High Reimbursement for Chemotherapy and Infusions

The majority of community oncology practice reimbursement comes in the form of noncognitive care. In 2006, the median oncologist's yearly salary was $358,000, the mean was $523,000, and the 90th percentile made over $1 million. Oncologists do not give chemotherapy just to make money, Dr. Smith said. According to one published study, reimbursement does not influence the decision to give chemotherapy or not, but the more generous the reimbursement the more expensive the chemotherapy oncologists use. For every dollar increase in reimbursement for the chemotherapy there is a $23 increase in overall chemotherapy costs (Jacobson et al., 2006). Throughout the last 10 years, oncology salaries have increased 86 percent while oncology visits have only increased 12 percent (Bodenheimer et al., 2007).

High-Income Expectations, Stress, and Burnout in Oncology

Oncologists have high-income expectations for doing their job. For many, it is a 24-hour-a-day, 7-day-a-week, 365-day-a-year responsibility to patient care. Furthermore, the looming 40 percent shortage of oncologists in this country will prevent any brisk reductions in salary in the near future. Within the current oncology payment structure, there is little reward for having a patient discussion on withholding chemotherapy because doing so is harder emotionally and will reduce reimbursement for the practice. Regarding our current incentives, Dr. Smith said:

> It is a lot easier and less angst producing to just give fourth-line chemotherapy than to sit with a 63-year-old guy with mesothelioma, as I did last Wednesday, and say "Your performance status is four," which he doesn't understand, "but you are in bed or the chair all the time. You are very short of breath. I know you desperately want to live longer, but there's no chemotherapy that has been shown in any randomized controlled trial … that is going to make you live longer or better. It would be different if you were much healthier." He is in tears. His wife is in tears. Three sons in the background are saying "Well, that's not what we read about on the Internet." Where's the reward for that? There isn't one except maybe doing a good job.

It is hard to take care of sick people. No one likes to break bad news. Add to that breaking bad financial news, and it becomes even more difficult (McFarlane et al., 2008). Dr. Smith said that he is very sympathetic to oncologists who would just give chemotherapy to please the family and patient, and give them some hope, rather than fight the uphill battle to get the patient into hospice at that point. There are no successful models for managing all of these expectations that oncologists have that do not require major shifts in lifestyle, incentives, and income.

Variable Quality of Care

The quality of cancer care is extremely variable, with many practices giving treatments that are not supported by evidence, such as fourth-, fifth-, or sixth-line chemotherapy for non-small cell lung cancer (NSCLC) or those with severely impaired functional status. Furthermore, the relative merits of treating actively versus hospice care are unclear. For instance, a recent study of Medicare beneficiaries with pancreatic and lung cancers enrolled in hospice found that those who received chemotherapy closer to their enrollment in hospice died sooner, consistent with death from side effects (Connor et al., 2007). This argues for early hospice referral, but there is no reward for oncologists who refer to hospice sooner, just lost income and difficult conversations. Lastly, there is little interest in performing non-inferiority trials to show treatment equivalency, though it could save society considerable amounts of money.

Potential Oncology Practice Solutions

Dr. Smith addressed each problem raised in the paragraphs above with specific suggestions to improve value in cancer practice.

Unrealistic or Uneducated Demands for Benefit

One thing we can do to reduce unrealistic expectations for cancer treatment benefit is revise the National Cancer Institute (NCI; www.cancer.gov) and American Cancer Society (ACS; www.cancer.org) websites to give truthful prognosis and treatment information to patients and their providers. Dr. Smith said that he and his colleagues were constructing an online resource for patients to show them data on prognosis with various treatment options in metastatic cancer. One example is shown in Figure 8-4. He explained that this information was not meant to dishearten patients, but to help them plan for all outcomes—cure or otherwise.

Consent forms for chemotherapy should ensure that oncologists consider and document their patient's Eastern Cooperative Oncology Group (ECOG) performance status (Oken et al., 1982), document his or her prognosis, specify the anticipated patient co-pay, specify the line of therapy planned, and specify the anticipated benefits and risks (Box 8-1). Insurance companies could then incentivize oncologists and patients who document these factors and then consider them in treatment decisions for

Breast cancer, fourth-line chemotherapy

What is my chance of being alive at 1 year if I take chemotherapy
or do best supportive care such as hospice? Without chemotherapy,
about 5 of 100 women would be alive at 1 year. With chemotherapy,
about 10 of 100 women would be alive at 1 year. The average woman
with breast cancer treated with "fourth-line chemotherapy " lived about
5 months. Half will do better, half worse.

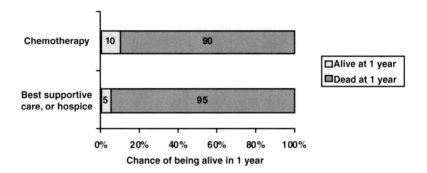

What is my chance of my being cured by chemotherapy?

FIGURE 8-4 Example of truthful patient information regarding metastatic cancer: fourth-line therapy for breast cancer.
SOURCE: Smith presentation, February 10, 2009; from GO8 NLM009525 Smith T (PI), Truthful Information about Prognosis and Options for People with Advanced Cancer.

third-, fourth-, or fifth-line treatments. However, criteria for decisions to limit treatment should be determined by society; doctors should not have to limit care in this way at the bedside without any external guidelines or support, Dr. Smith said.

Why bother bringing up discussions of death? Holly Prigerson's group prospectively followed several hundred patients who eventually died of their cancer (Wright et al., 2008). Only 37 percent of them ever had a discussion with their oncologists about the fact that they were dying from their cancer. She found that those 37 percent who were told that they were going to die from their cancer showed no difference in their mental health or worry, and were far less likely to want heroic measures, receive ventilation, or be admitted to the ICU. They were far more likely to admit being terminally ill, complete a do-not-resuscitate order, to use hospice, and to have opportunities for life review. In a companion article, the authors calculated the

BOX 8-1
Example Informational Consent Form for Treatment

I, _____ give _____ permission
to administer the following chemotherapy drugs to myself, _____

_____

I understand the risks of chemotherapy and have been provided
the following information:

( ) drug-specific information ( ) disease-specific information.

**I ( ) do ( ) do not want specific information about the
benefits of chemotherapy (see below).**

The goals of this therapy are (doctor should check the appropriate
area)
( ) cure
( ) to help me live longer (my disease is not likely to be cured)
( ) to help me feel better

Chemotherapy for my _____ cancer as 1st-, 2nd-, 3rd-,
4th-, _____-line treatment is expected to, on average:

- Increase my chance of being alive at 1 year from _____% to
  _____%
- Increase my survival compared to no treatment from _____
  months to _____months
- Prevent my cancer from getting worse (progressing) by
  _____months
- Shrink my cancer in half in ___ of 100 people like me
- Shrink my cancer completely in ___ of 100 people like me
- Keep my cancer stable for ___ months in ___ of 100 people
  like me
- Improve my cancer symptoms in ___ of 100 people like me

Patient signature: _____

MD signature: _____

Physician documentation of patient ECOG Performance Status,
0 to 4 (circle one):

      0 – no symptoms   **1** – symptoms but normal activity
         2 – symptoms but still functioning
         3 – in bed or chair ≤ 50% of the day
         4 – in bed or chair ≥ 50% of the day

costs of care for those who had the discussions were 36 percent lower than the cost for those who did not (Zhang et al., 2009). If one adds this to the 50 percent savings shown for switching from oncology services alone to oncology plus palliative care-based deaths in the hospital, the potential savings are considerable (Smith et al., 2003).

Low Reimbursement for Cognitive Care

Low reimbursement for cognitive care requires a significant revision of the current system toward rewarding good practice, not unsustainable entrepreneurship, said Dr. Smith. One solution could be paying all oncologists $50 per work-related RVU for cognitive care. Peter Eisenberg has gone so far as suggesting that oncology should be a salaried profession to reduce the incentive to administer inappropriate anticancer therapy (Eisenberg and Mahar, 2009). Alternatively, if payors think that having a nurse, chaplain, or psychologist is important, they could pay for these clinical staff directly, rather than through the oncologist's salary, Dr. Smith suggested. If these steps are taken beforehand, then profits from chemotherapy should be reduced, said Dr. Smith, one way or another.

High Reimbursement for Chemotherapy or Infusions and High-Income Expectations

We can reduce the incentives to overuse chemotherapy. Though it will be very complicated to develop capitated or illness-based episode payments, reimbursement could be reduced for chemotherapy to 6 percent over the average sales price. Furthermore, there should be a reward for oncologists who follow National Comprehensive Cancer Network (NCCN) guidelines (second-line NSCLC and third-line breast cancer) to switch to nonchemotherapy-based care when their patient's performance status reaches 3 or 4 (NCCN, 2009). Increasing government purchasing power to reduce the costs of drugs will be essential, and a U.S. version of the United Kingdom's National Institute of Health and Clinical Excellence (NICE) may be needed to assess the cancer drugs arriving soon from the pipeline.

Oncologists say they want to treat people, not disease, and these changes are all in line with that, Dr. Smith said. Oncologists in other countries seem reasonably happy and productive, Dr. Smith noted, and their patients' survival is the same.

Stress and Burnout

It is incredibly hard to take care of sick people. That is not going to change. In fact, Dr. Smith said, as people live longer—thank goodness—they have more complications. Dr. Smith emphasized that these difficulties should not be made worse by forcing oncologists to do the work of rationing that others (payors, government, society) avoid. Reasonable guidance and guidelines, clearly defined societal expectations, or the equivalent of a NICE are required to provide oncologists the decisions and support they need.

Variable Quality of Care

The American Society of Clinical Oncology's Quality Oncology Practice Initiative has successfully assessed oncology practices for adherence to published guidelines. Could this model be applied to assess the number of practices with appropriate counseling and social work staff? Could they be used to assess what percentage of practices delivers third-, fourth-, or higher-line chemotherapy, for which cancer types, and for patients at what performance status? Could they be used to track the percentage of practices that give chemotherapy or refer to hospice within the last 2 weeks of life? Dr. Smith said that all of these were achievable, but there was no reward for doing them—yet.

ADVOCATING FOR VALUE IN CANCER CARE

Ms. Ellen Stovall of the National Coalition for Cancer Survivorship said, with her 16 years of cancer-related advocacy in Washington, DC, she still believed that the job of citizen activists and advocates is to press for reforms and hold accountable the systems that organize health care, finance health care, finance cancer research, and regulate drug products in order to truly bring patient-centered care to people with cancer and their families. Cancer patients, for the most part, are treated outside any system of quality assurance or required accountability for cancer care. Many people diagnosed with cancer do not know that, and they may not want to know. They want to believe the care they receive is of value.

Everyone hopes for a cure for cancer. Every family wants this. Our society wants this. Our lawmakers want this. But we live in a society that is uncomfortable with something that we are all going to experience—our own death. The combination of our hope for a cure and our discomfort with mortality fails the patient and all those involved with their care. Research on thousands of cancer survivors over three decades shows that survivors fear pain and suffering, and they fear abandonment by their physicians and others. There is now a tremendous opportunity to ramp up discussions of retooling our cancer care system so that it is truly a patient-centered, health care delivery system that values and rewards participation in clinical research or registries, and so that it is a system that values the time health care professionals spend with patients by realigning reimbursement.

Clinicians also have the opportunity to promote the implementation of cancer treatment and survivorship plans that clearly spell out goals of treatment for each patient. This planning process would focus on treating the whole patient, not only the disease. Creating a cancer care plan after reviewing all the evidence-based choices available for treating each patient provides the foundation or framework for difficult, shared decision making. It also fosters a clinical relationship that is founded in openness and trust, telling the truth, and that values shared decisions, provides support and continuity of care, diminishes fear of abandonment, and accepts all visions of hope that patients and their family members bring to the treatment process.

Ms. Stovall concluded by saying that to achieve this vision of cancer care, FDA reform is needed to not only create novel ways of looking at clinical trial design but also to expand access to novel therapies. This should enable treatment knowledge to advance with every patient and provide equity and access to every patient. In addition, payment and financing reform are needed. This can be accomplished by working with private payors and Congress to realize Medicare reimbursement that values cancer care and survivorship care planning as fundamental elements of quality care. Finally, patient and physician education are needed, as well as close collaboration with those in the caregiving community to improve value in cancer care.

DISCUSSION

Dr. Newcomer asked Dr. Smith to clarify what he meant when he said in his presentation that physicians should not be making decisions about rationing at the bedside on an individual case-by-case basis. Is it not essential that physicians be in the discussion about where therapy should be stopped as a policy and at the bedside? Absolutely, said Dr. Smith, and he explained that oncologists and other physicians have a critical role to play in determining what works. Physicians are perhaps in the best position to make judgments about when to stop third- or fourth-line therapy.

What should not happen, however, is a situation in which physicians are forced to make decisions for individual patients at the bedside without the support of clinical guidelines or other decision makers who will back them up. Dr. Newcomer asked, who should be writing those rules? Dr. Smith said he believed it should be those involved in using the available health care funds. In the case of UnitedHealthcare, it is all of the patients covered. Dr. Tunis added that Dr. Newcomer's question at its core was asking, "Who should be responsible for rationing care?" It would be great if a U.S. NICE could remove the discomfort and burden of these decisions from all of us, but Dr. Tunis thought a U.S. NICE was unlikely in the near future. Dr. Chernew added that the fact that those paying into Medicare now are not the current beneficiaries introduces another difficulty in trying to decide who should be involved in rationing decisions. The current Medicare beneficiaries will tend to want Medicare to be much more aggressive than the younger people who are financing Medicare would want it to be. The same might be true of the majority of those paying premiums into private plans now who are not the minority spending the most on care through those plans.

Dr. Garrison asked whether NCCN and other guideline developers had a role to play. There was agreement among the panelists that American Society of Clinical Oncologists, NCCN, ACS, and NCI would all need to be involved in delivering truthful information to patients and clinicians about what can be done medically for their illnesses.

Mr. Merrill Goozner of the Center for Science in the Public Interest asked whether oncologists are being reimbursed for care that is unproven. Dr. Smith clarified and emphasized that oncologists are not giving unproven therapies, but they are administering therapy that is probably easier to give than having the very difficult discussions about prognosis and chance of cure. The difficulty also appears when helping people make decisions when their values are not shared by the clinicians guiding them. Clinicians providing guidance should be nondirective and help patients make tough decisions while holding an even keel.

Ms. Jennifer Hinkelfen of NCCN asked what role clinical practice guidelines have in helping to define what value is. Should cost considerations be implicit or explicit in the guidelines? Dr. Tunis responded by saying that it would be a very good idea to explicitly provide economic information on comparative costs of alternative treatments in the guidelines but perhaps not to integrate this fully into the clinical recommendations. In this format the information would be readily available to introduce it into the conversation, but not such that it would directly dictate clinical decisions.

Dr. Back suggested that a professional expectation be developed among oncologists that they engage and pursue these end-of-life conversations, guide trainees to do the same, and support one another to create a culture that makes this the norm. Dr. Smith agreed with the suggestion.

REFERENCES

Bodenheimer, T., R. A. Berenson, and P. Rudolf. 2007. The primary care–specialty income gap: Why it matters. *Annals of Internal Medicine* 146(4):301–306.

Chandra, A., J. Gruber, and R. McKnight. 2007. *Patient Cost-Sharing, Hospitalization Offsets, and the Design of Optimal Health Insurance for the Elderly.* Cambridge, MA: National Bureau of Economic Research.

Chernew, M. E., A. B. Rosen, and A. M. Fendrick. 2007. Value-based insurance design. *Health Affairs* 26(2):w195–w203.

Chernew, M. E., M. R. Shah, A. Wegh, S. N. Rosenberg, I. A. Juster, A. B. Rosen, M. C. Sokol, K. Yu-Isenberg, and A. M. Fendrick. 2008. Impact of decreasing copayments on medication adherence within a disease management environment: Value-based cost sharing can increase patients' adherence to important medications. *Health Affairs* 27(1):103–112.

Connor, S. R., B. Pyenson, K. Fitch, C. Spence, and K. Iwasaki. 2007. Comparing hospice and nonhospice patient survival among patients who die within a three-year window. *Journal of Pain and Symptom Managment* 33(3):238–246.

Cranor, C. W., B. A. Bunting, and D. B. Christensen. 2003. The Asheville Project: Long-term clinical and economic outcomes of a community pharmacy diabetes care program *Journal of the American Pharmaceutical Association* 43(5 Suppl):S36–S37.

Eisenberg, P., and M. Mahar. 2009. *A very open letter from an oncologist.* http://www.healthbeatblog.org/2009/01/a-very-open-letter-from-an-oncologist.html (accessed April 11, 2009).

Fendrick, A. M., D. G. Smith, M. E. Chernew, and S. N. Shah. 2001. A benefit-based copay for prescription drugs: Patient contribution based on total benefits, not drug acquisition cost. *American Journal of Managed Care* 7(9):861–867.

Freudenheim, M. 2007. To save later, some employers are offering free drugs now. *The New York Times,* February 21, 2007.

Fuhrmans, V. 2004. A radical prescription: While most companies look to slash health costs by shifting more expenses to employees, Pitney Bowes took a different tack. *The Wall Street Journal,* May 10, 2004.

Harrington, S. E., and T. J. Smith. 2008 The role of chemotherapy at the end of life: "When is enough, enough?" *Journal of the American Medical Association* 299(22):2667–2678.

Hillner, B., and T. J. Smith. 2009. Efficacy does not necessarily translate to cost effectiveness: A case study in the challenges associated with 21st-century cancer drug pricing. *Journal of Clinical Oncology* 27(13):2111–2113.

Jacobson, M., J. A. O'Malley, C. C. Earle, J. Pakes, P. Gaccione, and J. P. Newhouse. 2006. Does reimbursement influence chemotherapy treatment for cancer patients? *Health Affairs* 25(2):437–443.

Mahoney, J. J. 2005. Reducing patient drug acquisition costs can lower diabetes health claims. *American Journal of Managed Care* 11(5 Suppl):S170–S176.

McFarlane, J., J. Riggins, and T. J. Smith. 2008. SPIKE$: A six-step protocol for delivering bad news about the cost of medical care. *Journal of Clinical Oncology* 26(25):4200–4204.

Meropol, N. J., and K. A. Schulman. 2007. Cost of cancer: Issues and implications. *Journal of Clinical Oncology* 25(2):180–186.

NCCN (National Comprehensive Cancer Network). 2009. *National Comprehensive Cancer Network guidelines: Non-small-cell lung cancer and breast cancer.* http://www.nccn.org/professionals/physician_gls/f_guidelines.asp (accessed March 28, 2009).

Oken, M. M., R. H. Creech, D. C. Tormey, J. Horton, T. E. Davis, E. T. McFadden, and P. P. Carbone. 1982. Toxicity and response criteria of the Eastern Cooperative Group. *American Journal of Clinical Oncology* 5(6):649–655.

Siu, A. L., F. A. Sonnenberg, W. G. Manning, G. A. Goldberg, E. S. Bloomfield, J. P. Newhouse, and R. H. Brook. 1986. Inappropriate use of hospitals in a randomized trial of health insurance plans. *New England Journal of Medicine* 315(20):1259–1266.

Smith, T. J., P. Coyne, B. Cassel, L. Penberthy, A. Hopson, and M. A. Hager. 2003. A high-volume specialist palliative care unit and team may reduce in-hospital end-of-life care costs. *Journal of Palliative Medicine* 6(5):699–705.

Wilt, T. J., T. Shamliyan, B. Taylor, R. MacDonald, T. J., I. Rutks, K. Koeneman, C.-S. Cho, and R. L. Kane. 2008. *Comparative effectiveness of therapies for clinically localized prostate cancer: Comparative effectiveness review no. 13.* Rockville, MD: Agency for Healthcare Research and Quality.

Wright, A. A., B. Zhang, A. Ray, J. W. Mack, E. Trice, T. Balboni, S. L. Mitchell, V. A. Jackson, S. D. Block, P. K. Maciejewski, and H. G. Prigerson. 2008. Associations between end-of-life discussions, patient mental health, medical care near death, and caregiver bereavement adjustment. *Journal of the American Medical Association* 300(14):1665–1673.

Zhang, B., A. A. Wright, H. A. Huskamp, M. E. Nilsson, M. L. Maciejewski, C. C. Earle, S. D. Block, P. K. Maciejewski, and H. G. Prigerson. 2009. Health care costs in the last week of life: Associations with end of life conversations. *Archives of Internal Medicine* 169(5):480–488.

9

Toward a Shared Understanding
of Value

The final discussion of the workshop, Dr. Peter Bach of Memorial Sloan-Kettering Cancer Center explained, had two aims: First, all six moderators from the workshop's panels would provide a synthesis of the discussions they facilitated. Second, Dr. Bach extended an invitation to all the workshop attendees to synthesize what they had learned over the course of the workshop by raising key remaining questions, suggesting next steps, or proposing solutions for assessing and improving value in cancer care.

Dr. Bach began the discussion with his impressions of the workshop to that point. He emphasized that cancer is not a single disease but many different diseases, some with tremendous opportunity for cure and others with very little. These differences have implications for potential value-based insurance design for cancer therapies, he said. If value-based insurance design were applied to cancer care, patients would not be penalized financially just for being diagnosed with cancer. For therapies that are not effective, however, perhaps patients should be financially discouraged from pursuing them through value-based insurance structures. Promoting these changes through value-based insurance design in oncology could greatly improve value in the care delivered to cancer patients.

Dr. Bach reiterated another theme from the workshop—that many trials used for Food and Drug Administration (FDA) treatment approval produced too little information of use to payors, providers, or patients. The trials and their outcomes are not patient centered, and their narrow eligibility criteria make it difficult to apply findings to real-world populations, undercutting their ability to determine treatment effectiveness. To solve this problem, Dr. Bach asked, how can we develop evidence for cancer drug effectiveness after FDA approval?

On the theme of pharmaceutical pricing, Dr. Bach reviewed several approaches the workshop had discussed. Value-based pricing was one approach in which the price of a drug would be based on the health return of that drug, expressed in terms of cost per QALY, for instance. Another approach was the United Kingdom's NICE model with an explicit upper limit on cost per QALY to drive down prices. Coinsurance, or increased co-pays for more expensive or less effective drugs, came up a number of times as a way to sensitize patients to higher drug prices and drive manufacturers' prices down. Alternatively, a reimbursement-structured model, Dr. Bach said, would establish clinically-based drug interchangeability criteria to increase direct competition between drugs and manufacturers, interrupt the monopoly pricing structures manufacturers now benefit from, and drive down prices.

High coinsurance burden has ethical challenges, Dr. Bach said. If patient sensitivity to price varies as a result of different coinsurance rates, this may interfere with patient autonomy. There is no question that higher co-pays reduce utilization, and for tier-4 drugs with a coinsurance rate of 20 percent, the patients' financial disincentive can be on the order of thousands of dollars a month or tens of thousands of dollars a year. An intriguing question, Dr. Bach said, was whether the financial burden of the co-pay poses an ethical risk to autonomy, or the simple presence of coinsurance of any size is enough to be ethically problematic.

Lastly, Dr. Bach reiterated the theme that clinicians at the bedside should not be expected to ration care on their own, especially in cases when their patients may benefit from treatments with extraordinarily high costs. Dr. Bach had concerns about putting clinicians in this role—given that clinicians' ability to provide evidence-based care has been uneven at best, should they be solely responsible for limiting care at the bedside? The reality is that clinicians have a strong independent streak and feel that they should be autonomous decision makers, and they are unlikely to accept external pressures to ration care.

Dr. Bach then turned to the panel of moderators for their comments.

WORKSHOP MODERATOR PERSPECTIVES

Clinician–Patient Communication and Its Influence on Value

About 80 percent of cancer patients in this country are treated in the community, where physicians are feeling considerable strain and salaries are declining, said Dr. Lichter. The landscape of oncology is going to change as a result, and those of us in the oncology community will have to decide whether we want to sit back and let that happen or be more assertive, envision the oncology system we want for our patients, and then help create it.

The first panel talked about communication, Dr. Lichter said, and it would be hard to find a topic more pertinent to value in cancer care, or one with greater potential to affect value in the near term. We can all communicate better. Communication is a learned skill that all of us, trainees and experienced practitioners alike, can continually improve upon. Ultimately these skills should be used to better engage in end-of-life discussions, set realistic goals, and communicate truthfully and openly with patients.

At ASCO, we want to play our role, Dr. Lichter said. The ASCO Cost of Care Task Force has been working for a year; learning modules to improve physician communication skills are being developed, and informational materials have been made available to help physicians and patients engage in difficult conversations about costs of care. The Quality Oncology Practice Initiative has the ability to measure many of the outcomes relevant to cancer care value through the 400 practices it tracks, and this data could be used to benchmark best practices and drive improvement in oncologists' performance on a large scale through self-correction among academics and the community oncologists alike. Dr. Lichter also said that ASCO, working with the NCCN, would continue to actively develop clear practice guidelines not just for early-stage cancer but late-stage disease as well.

Lastly, oncology is a natural fit for value-based insurance design, Dr. Lichter said. Clearly, the co-pay for highly effective treatments such as trastuzumab, which reduces a patient's chance of recurrence by 50 percent, should not be the same as the co-pay for the least effective fifth-line therapy. This is an area where progress can be made.

Generating Evidence About Effectiveness and Value

Many dimensions of value have been covered at this workshop, Dr. Cohen said. His panel, he explained, approached value in terms of outcomes and effectiveness. Dr. Woodcock's presentation elucidated the ways in which drug efficacy and safety were established through the FDA approval process. A challenge that remained for the FDA was to incorporate patient-specific outcome measures, among other challenges. In his presentation, Dr. Sargent posed the challenge of predicting effectiveness from efficacy, citing limitations of RCTs and the utility of large-scale observational studies. Cost was largely absent from this panel's discussion, Dr. Cohen explained. In fact, Dr. Woodcock made it clear that cost-effectiveness analysis did not factor into the FDA's drug approval process at all.

Value and the Oncology Market

The speakers in Dr. Lerner's panel, he said, discussed the poor incentive structures in oncology, the numerous constituencies to be taken into account when pharmaceutical manufacturers price a drug, and the barriers to generating meaningful cost-effectiveness data in clinical trials. Reflecting on the workshop as a whole, Dr. Lerner added that the cancer care community should provide better evidence-based information directly to patients, whether through informed consent or other routes. The solutions for improving value in cancer care are unlikely to come from within the professions with all of its competing goals, Dr. Lerner said. Instead, informing patients and empowering them with a different role in their care could be much more productive.

Value in Cancer Practice: Health Insurer Perspectives

Oncologists are like the rest of us, Dr. Ramsey said. They are like other physicians too, whether in primary care or other specialties. Speaking as a primary care physician, Dr. Ramsey said we all want value-based health care and we all want to consider the impacts of health care decisions on society's shared resources, but we are conflicted when faced with the patient in front of us who is in need and we want to help. As a result, most physicians' cost-effectiveness thresholds are probably higher than they or economists would like.

Cost-effectiveness seems to be health care's "third rail" in the United States—no one will touch it. Why then is the use of cost-effectiveness so well-accepted in Europe? While there may be interest groups and policy makers who would like to avoid considering cost-effectiveness in this country, Dr. Ramsey thought that we were ready as a society to confront costs in health care, and understanding cost-effectiveness would be a transparent way to begin the discussion. Lastly, Dr. Ramsey reiterated that there is considerable variation in oncology practice, and reducing this variation from the moment a patient is diagnosed with cancer seems a logical target for the cancer community's efforts.

Ethical Issues for Value-Based Decision Making in Oncology

Dr. Moses reiterated suggestions from the speakers on his panel. One need that was presented, he said, was a willingness to ration last-chance care at the end of life. He also emphasized the need for oncologists to better inform patients and participate in care decisions at the end of life.

Improving Value in Oncology: Ways Forward

Since our current national health reform discussion is focusing on universal coverage, it tends to overlook the related issues of cost and coordination. Yet much of the discussion at this workshop has been about costs and coordination of care near the end of life of cancer patients, Dr. Garrison said. The U.S. health care system has often been called a "blank check" health care system in that those of us who have excellent private health insurance are able to receive any care for which we expect a marginal positive health benefit, regardless of the societal marginal cost, Dr. Garrison said. This incentive for socially inefficient use underlies our high share of medical spending and its high growth rate. Dr. Garrison asked: How will we help oncologists constrain costs or support their treatment decisions in cases where the potential for a marginal clinical benefit exists but it is small relative to the marginal costs? That is the challenge. The tools of cost-effectiveness analysis can help us to address these trade-offs, thereby addressing the value question.

What do we mean by value? Dr. Garrison said that he was comfortable describing value from an economic perspective as cost-effectiveness. But there were other types of value that emerged during the workshop that need to be included in the calculus for value in cancer care. There is value to patients in having an opportunity for treatment benefit, in reducing uncertainty through better information, and in personalizing medicine, Dr. Garrison asserted. These types of value are not normally included in the calculation of cost-effectiveness, but they are important benefits that should be measured and considered.

GROUP DISCUSSION OF VALUE IN CANCER CARE

Workshop Attendee Perspectives

Building on Dr. Rossi's presentation, Dr. Ganz concluded that the price that pharmaceutical manufacturers choose at the launch of a drug may not be the appropriate price once it has been studied in a larger population or earlier in the course of disease. While drug prices at launch may be too high for their survival benefit, if the drug is very valuable when studied in larger populations, pharmaceutical manufacturers should not be penalized and forced to set artificially low initial prices. Dr. Ganz proposed that creative solutions be sought to address this problem of dynamic pricing in oncology, which could help avoid drugs with such high prices at launch while assuring that drugs are priced according to benefits throughout their life cycle.

Dr. Ganz also suggested that some mechanism be developed to collect data on outcomes of therapies paid for by insurance plans by using the data those plans already collect. Perhaps pharmaceutical manufacturers, the Centers for Medicare and Medicaid Services (CMS), or some other funder could support this research to benefit the overall societal good. This could be a way to do large-scale studies without concerns over whether those with vested interests (manufacturers, clinical researchers, etc.) would provide support, and it could deliver large amounts of real-world information.

Dr. Murphy raised a number of points contrasting pediatric oncology with adult oncology. In pediatric oncology, she said, treatment tends to be protocol-based to a greater extent, and few patients are treated in the community. Also, most pediatric oncologists are salaried. If adult oncologists were also paid on a salary structure, this could remove remunerative conflicts of interest that drive provision of fifth- or sixth-line chemotherapy with little effectiveness.

Dr. Chernew commented on the distinction between those patients who pay a significant price for care that benefits them and those who pay the same price for futile treatment. Ethically, the fundamental problem is not that the latter patients are charged high prices for futile treatment—it is that they are encouraged to pursue the futile treatment at all. Dr. Chernew tied this to a second point on the need for broader, systems-level research into the structures and incentives in place that encourage physicians to practice in the ways that they do.

Dr. Vikram said that the NCI had in the past funded a wide variety of projects in addition to research, from guidelines development to building public awareness, but the shrinking NCI budget had curtailed the scope of its work. With a mandate from Congress and greater funding, Dr. Vikram was confident that the National Institutes of Health, and NCI in particular, could expand its role to include research in areas relevant to value in cancer care, such as comparative effectiveness or research to help oncologists make decisions at the bedside.

ATTRIBUTES AND METRICS OF VALUE IN CANCER CARE

Dr. Ramsey invited all those in attendance at the workshop to consider and comment on attributes of value in cancer care and metrics for measuring value. Synthesizing common themes from the workshop, he presented a list of attributes and metrics of value in cancer care, as well as stakeholder perspectives to be considered (Table 9-1). Were there things missing from these lists, Dr. Ramsey asked the audience, or things that should not be included?

Hope should be added as an attribute of value, said Dr. Ganz.

Social equity should be added as an attribute of value, said Dr. Smith.

Another participant suggested adding the public at large or a societal perspective to the list of stakeholder perspectives, as well as adverse events associated with treatment to the value attributes.

Variation in care and standardization through compliance with guidelines should be added as a metric, said Dr. Moses.

Mr. John Frick of the Blue Cross and Blue Shield Association suggested that the metrics of value should include the number of generic biologics available in the marketplace.

Dr. Ganz suggested coordination of care as a value metric.

At the end of this discussion and the workshop overall, the list of value metrics, attributes, and stakeholder perspectives included all those listed in Table 9-1.

TABLE 9-1 Proposed Value Attributes, Value Metrics, and Stakeholder Perspectives

Attributes of Value	Metrics of Value	Pertinent Stakeholder Perspectives
Outcome Attributes	Economic Metrics	Patient perspective, including families or other social supports
Survival—duration of life	Cost per QALY	Physician or clinician perspective
Quality of life	Equity Metrics	Health insurer perspective—public and private
Adverse events	Variation in care	Pharmaceutical manufacturer perspective
Time to progression	Financial hardship	Societal perspective—the public at large
Tumor response	Workforce or service shortages	
Cost	Access to insurance and appropriate services	
Care Attributes	Disparities in care	
Access to care	Innovation Metrics	
Quality of care	Willingness to pay for cancer treatment research	
Communication	FDA new drug applications	
Social equity	Generic treatments	
Patient-Centered Attributes	Biosimilars	
Compassion and respect	Care Metrics	
Opportunity for treatment benefit	Quality of clinician–patient communication	
Choice	Coordination of care	
Hope		
Innovation and Future Discovery		

SOURCE: Ramsey presentation, February 10, 2009.

Acronyms

ACS   American Cancer Society
ASCO   American Society of Clinical Oncology
ASP   average sales price
ATC4   anatomical therapeutic classification
AWP   average wholesale price

CCDR   Canadian Coordinated Drug Review
CED   coverage with evidence development
CMS   Centers for Medicare and Medicaid Services

FDA   U.S. Food and Drug Administration

GDP   gross domestic product

HTA   health technology assessment

ICD   implantable cardiac defibrillator
ICER   incremental cost-effectiveness ratio
IND   investigational new drug
IOM   Institute of Medicine

NCCN   National Comprehensive Cancer Network
NCI   National Cancer Institute
NCPF   National Cancer Policy Forum
NHS   National Health Service (United Kingdom)
NICE   U.K. National Institute for Health and Clinical Excellence
NIH   National Institutes of Health
NSCLC   non-small cell lung cancer

PBM   pharmacy benefit manager
PhRMA   Pharmaceutical Research and Manufacturers of America

QALY   quality-adjusted life-year

RCT   randomized controlled trial
RVU   relative value unit

VBID   value-based insurance design

Glossary

Accelerated Approval—the process by which the FDA rapidly approves experimental treatments for serious or life-threatening conditions, often based on data using surrogate endpoints.

Advance Care Planning—involves taking the time to learn and discuss end-of-life care options and services before a health crisis, then making choices based on a person's priorities, beliefs and values and sharing his or her wishes in writing through an *advance directive.*

Anatomical Therapeutic Classification (ATC)—used for the classification of drugs, this system divides drugs into different groups according to the organ or system on which they act and/or their therapeutic and chemical characteristics.

Bevacizumab (Avastin)—a monoclonal antibody drug used to treat metastatic cancer of the colon and rectum, usually in combination with 5-fluorouracil-basd chemotherapy. Bevacizumab is also used in the treatment of advanced, recurrent, or metastatic non-squamous non-small cell lung cancer, in combination with carboplatin and paclitaxel, or other cancer drugs, and metastatic HER2-negative breast cancer, in combination with paclitaxel.

Biomarker—a biochemical substance found in blood, other body fluids, or tissues used as an indicator of a biologic state that is objectively measured and evaluated as an indicator of normal biologic processes, pathogenic processes, or a response to therapeutic intervention.

Bortezomib (Velcade)—a drug approved in the United States for treating relapsed multiple myeloma and mantle cell lymphoma. NICE recommended against use of bortezomib in 2006.

Cancer registry—a system that monitors cancer cases that have been diagnosed or treated in one institution or a specific geographic area.

Cetuximab (Erbitux)—a monoclonal antibody drug used to treat advanced or metastatic cancer of the colon and rectum, usually in combination with chemotherapy or irinotecan, another cancer drug.

Clinical endpoint—a characteristic or variable that reflects how a patient feels, functions, or survives in response to a medical intervention.

Clinical practice guidelines—systematically defined statements to assist practitioner and patient decisions about appropriate health care for specific clinical circumstances.

Clinical trial—a formal study carried out according to a prospectively defined protocol that is intended to discover or verify the safety and effectiveness of procedures or interventions in humans.

Cluster randomization—the randomization of groups (or clusters) of subjects. May be used as a randomization strategy in clinical trials.

Cohort study—an observational study in which outcomes in a group of patients that received an intervention are compared with outcomes in a similar group, that is, the cohort, either contemporary or historical, of patients that did not receive the intervention.

Coinsurance—the percentage of medical care costs covered by an insured individual beyond the deductible. In many cases, coinsurance is paid by the insured individual until a predefined limit is reached, after which all costs are covered by the health care plan. Coinsurance also is used to refer to supplemental insurance used to pay the fees not covered by the primary health care plan. Coinsurance is often synonymous with co-payment.

Colectomy—excision of a portion of the colon or its entirety (open vs. laparoscopic-assisted).

Co-payment or co-pay—the percentage of medical care costs covered by an insured individual beyond the deductible. Co-payment is often shortened to "co-pay," and may be synonymous with coinsurance (see Coinsurance above).

Cost-effectiveness—the degree to which a service or a medical treatment meets a specified goal at an acceptable cost and level of quality. Cost-effectiveness analysis is a comparison of alternative interventions in which costs are measured in monetary units and outcomes are measured in non-monetary units, e.g., reduced mortality or morbidity.

Cost sharing—a general set of financing arrangements via deductibles, co-pays and/or coinsurance in which a person covered by the health plan must pay some of the costs to receive care.

Coverage with Evidence Development (CED)—a CMS program whereby prospective data collection on a product is required for national Medicare coverage. A product that has an insufficient evidence base for CMS coverage determination could be evaluated through CED.

Do-not-resuscitate (DNR) order—a document that informs medical personnel not to attempt a resuscitation in the event of a patient's cardiac or respiratory arrest. The order is written after a discussion with the patient, family, or designated surrogate decision maker. Also called a do-not-attempt resuscitation (DNAR) order.

Effectiveness—how well a treatment works in practice.

Efficacy—the capacity for producing a desired result or effect under ideal conditions, for example, in a laboratory setting or within the protocol of a carefully managed randomized controlled trial.

End-of-life care—the care provided to a person in their final stages of life.

Erlotinib (Tarceva)—a drug used to treat locally advanced or metastatic non-small cell lung cancer and other cancers. It targets epidermal growth factor receptor tyrosine kinase, and specific genetic mutations correlate to patients' response to the drug.

FDA premarket approval—FDA approval for a new drug or device that enables it to be marketed for clinical use. To receive this approval, the manufacturer of the product must submit clinical data showing the product is safe and effective for its intended use.

Functional status—a measure of an individual's ability to perform normal activities of life. Encompasses a wide variety of patient-focused outcomes including physical functioning, emotional well-being, and social functioning.

Health technology assessment (HTA)—the systematic evaluation of properties, effects, and/or impacts of health care technology. It may address the direct, intended consequences of technologies as well as their indirect, unintended consequences. Its main purpose is to inform technology-related policy making in health care. HTA is conducted by interdisciplinary groups using explicit analytical frameworks drawing from a variety of methods.

Hospice—a discrete site of care in the form of an inpatient hospital or nursing home unit or a free-standing facility; an organization or program that provides, arranges, and advises on a wide range of medical and supportive services for dying patients and their families and friends; an approach to care for dying patients based on clinical, social, and metaphysical or spiritual principles.

Hospitalist—a physician specializing in hospital inpatient care.

Human epidermal growth factor receptor 2 (HER2)—a growth factor receptor that is used as a breast cancer biomarker for prognosis and treatment with the drug trastuzumab (Herceptin), which targets the protein.

Implantable cardiac defibrillator (ICD)—a surgically implanted electronic device capable of sending an electric shock to the heart to stop an extremely rapid, irregular heartbeat and restore the normal heart rhythm.

Intention to treat analysis—a type of analysis of clinical trial data in which all patients are included in the analysis based on their original assignment to intervention or control groups, regardless of whether patients failed to fully participate in the trial for any reason, including whether they actually received their allocated treatment, dropped out of the trial, or crossed over to another group.

Laparoscopy or laparoscopic-assisted surgery—a type of surgical procedure in which a small incision is made through which a viewing tube (laparoscope) is inserted. The laparoscope contains a small camera on the eyepiece, allowing the surgeon to examine the abdominal and pelvic organs on a video monitor. Other small incisions can be made to insert instruments to perform procedures. Laparoscopy is less invasive than regular, open abdominal surgery.

Large, simple trial—prospective, randomized controlled trials that use large numbers of patients, broad patient inclusion criteria, multiple study sites, minimal data requirements, and electronic registries; their purposes include detecting small and moderate treatment effects, gaining effectiveness data, and improving external validity.

Medicare—a public health care program for individuals aged 65 and older, those who have permanent kidney failure, and people with certain disabilities. It includes Part A for coverage of hospitalization-related expenses, Part B for coverage of medical care, and Part D for prescription drug coverage. Part C, sometimes called a Medicare Advantage

Plan, is a combination of Part A and Part B but the coverage is provided through private insurance companies approved by Medicare.

Metastasis—spread of cancer from its original anatomical site to one or more additional body sites.

Moral hazard—the prospect that a person insulated from risk may behave differently than he or she would behave if fully exposed to the risk.

Off-label use—use of a drug that either has not been approved by the FDA or has not been approved for the purpose for which it is being used.

Palliative care—treatment of symptoms associated with the effects of cancer and its treatment, with a focus on reducing pain and suffering and improving quality of life.

Panitumumab (Vectibix)—a monoclonal antibody drug used to treat metastatic colon cancer expressing the epidermal growth factor receptor.

Pharmacy benefit manager (PBM)—an administrator of prescription drug programs, primarily responsible for processing and paying prescription drug claims. A PBM is also responsible for developing and maintaining the formulary, contracting with pharmacies, and negotiating discounts and rebates with drug manufacturers.

Phase I trial—clinical trial in a small number of patients in which the toxicity and optimal dosing of an intervention are assessed.

Phase II trial—clinical trial in which the safety and preliminary efficacy of an intervention are assessed in patients.

Phase III trial—large-scale clinical trial in which the safety and efficacy of an intervention are assessed in a large number of patients (sometimes divided into Phase IIIa trials conducted before regulatory submission and Phase IIIb trials conducted after regulatory submission but before approval).

Phase IV trial—postmarketing study to monitor long-term effects and provide additional information on safety and efficacy, including for different regimens and patient groups.

Price elasticity—measures how much the quantity or supply of a good, or demand for it, changes if its price changes. If the percentage change in quantity is more than the percentage change in price, the good is price elastic; if it is less, the good is inelastic.

Price sensitivity—the extent to which price is an important criterion in the customer's decision-making process.

Quality-adjusted life-year (QALY)—a unit of health care outcomes that adjusts gains (or losses) in years of life subsequent to a health care intervention by the quality of life during those years. QALYs can provide a common unit for comparing cost-effectiveness across different interventions and health problems. Analogous units include disability-adjusted life-years (DALYs) and healthy-years equivalents (HYEs).

Randomized controlled trial (RCT)—a true prospective experiment in which investigators randomly assign an eligible sample of patients to one or more treatment groups and a control group and follow patients' outcomes (also known as a randomized clinical trial).

Relative value unit (RVU)—a comparable service measure used to permit comparison of the amounts of resources required to perform various health care services. It is determined by assigning weight to such factors as personnel time, level of skill, and sophistication of equipment required to render patient services.

Response rate—the percentage of patients in whom treatment results in a significant change in the clinical endpoint of interest.

Standardized patient—an individual who is trained to act as a real patient in order to simulate a set of symptoms or problems.

Statistical power—the probability of detecting a treatment effect of a given magnitude when a treatment effect of at least that magnitude truly exists.

Surrogate endpoint—a biomarker that is intended to substitute for a clinical endpoint in a therapeutic clinical trial and is expected to predict clinical benefit (or lack thereof) based on epidemiologic, therapeutic, pathophysiologic, or other scientific evidence.

Time to tumor progression (progression-free survival)—the time interval from the start of treatment to cancer progression. It is a measure of the clinical benefit from therapy.

Trastuzumab (Herceptin)—see HER2.

Value-based insurance design—a system of patient coinsurance based on the value—not simply the price—of health care services.

Appendix A

Workshop Agenda

Assessing and Improving Value in Cancer Care
A National Cancer Policy Forum Workshop

Monday and Tuesday, February 9 and 10, 2009
NAS Lecture Room
National Academy of Sciences Building
2100 C Street, NW
Washington, DC

DAY ONE

8:00 a.m. **Welcome, Introductory Remarks: What Is Value in Cancer Care? Why Is It Important?**
Scott D. Ramsey, *Fred Hutchinson Cancer Research Center*

8:20 **Physician–Patient Communication and Its Influence on Value**
Moderator: Allen S. Lichter, *American Society of Clinical Oncology*

8:25 **Inside the Physician–Patient Discussion in Cancer Care**
Speaker: Anthony Back, *University of Washington*

8:55 Invited Comments from Diane Blum, CancerCare

9:00 **Can We Communicate Effectively with Cancer Patients About the Benefits and Risks of Cancer Treatments?**
Speaker: Peter A. Ubel, *University of Michigan*

9:30 Invited Comments from Mary McCabe, *Memorial Sloan-Kettering Cancer Survivorship Program*

9:35 **Therapy for Advanced-Stage Cancer: What Do Patients Want and Expect?**
Speaker: Robert Erwin, *Marti Nelson Cancer Foundation*

10:05 Invited Comments from Ellen Stovall, *National Coalition for Cancer Survivorship*

10:10 Discussion

10:40 **10-Minute Break**

10:50 **Generating Evidence About Effectiveness and Value**
Moderator: Steven B. Cohen, *Agency for Healthcare Research and Quality*

10:55 **FDA Perspectives on Evidence for Regulatory Approval in Cancer**
Speaker: Janet Woodcock, *Food and Drug Administration*

11:25 **What Constitutes Reasonable Evidence of Efficacy and Effectiveness?**
Speaker: Daniel J. Sargent, *Mayo Clinic*

11:55 Discussion

12:25 p.m. **Lunch**

1:00 **Value and the Oncology Market**
Moderator: Jeffrey C. Lerner, *ECRI Institute*

1:05 **Drug Pricing and Value in Oncology vs. Other Areas in Medicine**
Speaker: Patricia M. Danzon, *University of Pennsylvania*

1:35 **Industry Perspective on Pharmaceutical Pricing in Oncology**
Speaker: Greg Rossi, *Genentech, Inc.*

2:05   Cost Implications: Strategies to Enhance Value in
        Oncology
        Speaker: Deborah Schrag, *Dana-Farber/Harvard Cancer
        Center*

        2:35 Discussion

3:20   10-Minute Break

3:30   Value in Cancer Practice: Health Insurer Perspectives
        Moderator: Scott D. Ramsey, *Fred Hutchinson Cancer
        Research Center*

3:35   Oncologists' Perception of Value in Oncology
        Speaker: Peter J. Neumann, *Tufts Medical Center*

4:05   Paying for New Cancer Treatments: Rights and
        Responsibilities of Health Insurers
        Speaker: Lee Newcomer, *United Healthcare*

4:35   European Experience and Perspectives on Evaluating
        Value for Oncology Products
        Speaker: Michael Drummond, *Centre for Health Economics,
        University of York*

        5:05 Discussion

5:50   Adjourned for the day

                        DAY TWO

8:00 a.m. Ethical Issues for Value-Based Decision Making in
           Oncology
           Moderator: Harold L. Moses, *Vanderbilt-Ingram Cancer
           Center*

8:05   Ethical Issues When Considering Insurance Coverage
           Based on Value in the Treatment of Cancer
           Speaker: Dan W. Brock, *Harvard Medical School*

8:35   **Patient–Physician Communication on Therapy Options for Cancer: Ethical Issues**
Speaker: Neil S. Wenger, *University of California, Los Angeles*

9:05 Discussion

9:35   **10-Minute Break**

9:45   **Improving Value in Oncology Practice: Ways Forward**
Moderator: Lou Garrison, *University of Washington*

9:50   **Value-Based Insurance Design—Initiatives Outside of Oncology**
Speaker: Michael Chernew, *Harvard Medical School*

10:20   **Generating Evidence of Value Post-FDA Approval: Is There a Role for Health Insurers?**
Speaker: Sean R. Tunis, *Center for Medical Technology Policy*

10:50   **Are There Ways to Improve the Value of Cancer Care That May Work at the Bedside?**
Speaker: Thomas J. Smith, *Virginia Commonwealth University*

11:20 Discussion

WORKING LUNCH

12:05 p.m. **Toward a Shared Understanding of Value: Can We Agree, and Does Perspective Matter?**
Moderator: Peter Bach, *Memorial Sloan-Kettering Cancer Center*
Panel: All Moderators

1:30   **Meeting Adjourned**

Appendix B

Speaker and Moderator Biographies

Scott D. Ramsey, M.D., Ph.D. (*Chair*), is a Full Member in the Cancer Prevention Program, Division of Public Health Science at the Fred Hutchinson Cancer Research Center. He directs the Cancer Technology Assessment Group, a multidisciplinary team devoted to clinical and economic evaluations of new and existing cancer prevention, screening, and treatment technologies. In addition, Dr. Ramsey is a Professor in the School of Medicine, School of Pharmacy, and the Institute for Public Health Genetics at the University of Washington. He is a member of the Institute of Medicine's National Cancer Policy Forum. Dr. Ramsey's research focuses on economic evaluations in cancer. He has published widely on patterns of care, costs, and cost-effectiveness of treatments for lung, colorectal, and prostate cancer. His current studies—funded by the National Cancer Institute, National Human Genome Research Institute, Centers for Disease Control and Prevention, and several pharmaceutical manufacturers—include projects to develop a genetic screening policy model for colorectal cancer, a multicenter study of decision making for men with newly diagnosed prostate cancer, and studies of cancer screening, incidence, treatment, and outcomes for Native Americans diagnosed with cancer. Along with investigators at the University of Washington, Dr. Ramsey codirects an NCI-funded training program in biobehavioral and cancer outcomes research.

Peter Bach, M.D., MAPP, is a member of the Health Outcomes Research Group in the Department of Epidemiology and Biostatistics, and a pulmonary and critical care physician in the Department of Medicine at Memorial Sloan-Kettering Cancer Center. His main research interests are in assessing and improving the quality of cancer care. His work has focused particularly on improving the quality of care for African American patients in Medicare, including cancer care. His work has shown that low quality of care contributes to excess mortality for African Americans with lung cancer, and that limited access to high-quality primary care physicians may reduce quality of care more generally for African Americans. He also studies the link between cigarette smoking, lung cancer, and early detection, and has developed statistical models that can be used to predict the probability that someone will develop lung cancer based on their age and smoking history. These models were recently used to demonstrate that CT screening for lung cancer may not benefit patients: people who are screened appear to die of lung cancer at the same rate as if they had not been screened, despite CT screening detecting many early lung cancers and leading to many diagnostic tests, invasive procedures, and surgeries. Dr. Bach is also engaged in health care policy work. In 2005 and 2006 he served as Senior Adviser to the Administrator of the Centers for Medicare and Medicaid Services (CMS) in Washington, DC, where he oversaw the agency's cancer initiatives, evidence development work through conditional coverage, and data policy. In that role, he was a liaison to other health agencies, including the FDA, NIH, and AHRQ. He currently serves as a member of the Institute of Medicine's National Cancer Policy Forum. He is the recipient of the Boyer award for clinical research, was the previous incumbent of the Frederick Adler faculty chair, and has been the recipient of grants from the National Cancer Institute, the National Institute of Aging, and the American Lung Association. Dr. Bach is a graduate of Harvard College, the University of Minnesota Medical School, and the University of Chicago School for Public Policy. He conducted his medical residency and subspecialty fellowship at the Johns Hopkins Hospital in Baltimore, Maryland. During the 1994 Rwandan civil war, he provided medical care to refugees in Goma, Zaire.

Anthony Back, M.D., is Professor of Medicine at the University of Washington in Seattle. He is Director of the Cancer Communication and Palliative Care Programs at the Seattle Cancer Care Alliance and the Fred Hutchinson Cancer Research Center. He is a board-certified medical oncologist whose primary research interests are physician–patient communication and palliative care, and he practices gastrointestinal oncology. Dr. Back was a Faculty Scholar on the Project on Death in America and is a member of the ASCO Communication Task Force. He is the Principal Investigator for the Oncotalk Teach, communication skills training program for Medical Oncology fellows (R25 CA 119019), and is an investigator on other NIH-funded observational studies of physician–patient communication about hope and information (R01 PI J.R. Curtis) and prognosis in hematologic malignancies (R01 P.I. Stephanie Lee).

Diane S. Blum, M.S.W., is Executive Director of CancerCare, Inc., a national nonprofit organization that provides free professional support services including counseling, education, financial assistance and practical help to people with cancer and their loved ones. Ms. Blum joined CancerCare in 1984 as Director of Social Service, and became Executive Director in 1990. Previously, Ms. Blum served as a social work supervisor at Memorial Sloan-Kettering Cancer Center and the Dana Farber Cancer Institute. Ms. Blum's areas of expertise include the psychosocial needs of cancer patients and their families, costs of cancer treatments and care, women and breast cancer, cancer survivorship, and nonprofit management. Cofounder of the National Alliance of Breast Cancer Organizations, Ms. Blum is also a founder of National Breast Cancer Awareness Month and serves as Editor-in-Chief of cancer.net, the ASCO website for patients and the public. She is also a member of the editorial boards of five other oncology-related publications. Additionally, she has served on committees of the Institute of Medicine, ASCO, and the National Association of Social Work, among others. Most recently, Ms. Blum was one of 15 members of an expert panel that recommended psychosocial services be included as standard care for all cancer patients. She currently serves on ASCO's Cost of Care Task Force, examining the financial impact of cancer treatments on patients and their families. Ms. Blum's awards include the Lifetime Achievement Award from the Board of Sponsors of National Breast Cancer Awareness Month, the Special Recognition Award from the National Coalition for Cancer Survivorship, the Republic Bank Breast Cancer Research Foundation Award, and the Special Recognition Award of the American Society of Clinical Oncology. Ms. Blum has written and lectured extensively about the psychosocial needs of cancer patients and their families. Her research has been published in a variety of medical journals including the *American Journal of Hospice and Palliative Care, Journal of Oncology, Journal of Psychosocial Oncology, Journal of Pain and Symptom Management, Annals of Internal Medicine,* and *Oncology Nursing News,* among others. Ms. Blum received a bachelor's degree from the University of Rochester and a master's degree from the School of Social Welfare at the State University of New York at Buffalo.

Dan W. Brock, Ph.D., is the Frances Glessner Lee Professor of Medical Ethics in the Department of Social Medicine, the Director of the Division of Medical Ethics at the Harvard Medical School, and the Director of the Harvard University Program in Ethics and Health. Prior to his arrival at Harvard, Professor Brock was Senior Scientist and a member of the Department of Clinical Bioethics at the National Institutes of Health. Until July 2002, he was Charles C. Tillinghast, Jr., University Professor, Professor of Philosophy and Biomedical Ethics, and Director of the Center for Biomedical Ethics at Brown University where he had a joint appointment in the Philosophy Department (of which he was Chair from 1980 to 1986) and in the Medical School. He served as Staff Philosopher on the President's Commission for the Study of Ethical Problems in Medicine in 1981–1982, and in 1993 was a member of the Ethics Working Group of the Clinton Task Force on National Health Reform. He has been a consultant in biomedical ethics and health policy to numerous national and international bodies, including the Office of Technology Assessment of the U.S. Congress, the Institute of Medicine, the National Bioethics Advisory Commission, and the World Health Organization. He is a Fellow and former member of the Board of Directors of the Hastings Center, and was a Fellow in the Ethics and Professions' Program and in the Division of Medical Ethics at Harvard University in 1991–1992. He was President of the American Association of Bioethics in 1995–1996, and was a founding Board Member of the American Society for Bioethics and Humanities. He is the author of over 150 articles in bioethics and in moral and political philosophy, which have appeared in books and refereed scholarly journals, including the *New England Journal of Medicine, JAMA, Science, Hastings Center Report, Philosophy and Public Affairs*, and *Ethics*. He is the author of *Deciding for Others: The Ethics of Surrogate Decision Making*, 1989, (with Allen E. Buchanan); *Life and Death: Philosophical Essays in Biomedical Ethics*, 1993; and *From Chance to Choice: Genetics and Justice* (with Allen Buchanan, Norman Daniels, and Daniel Wikler), 2000, all published by Cambridge University Press. He is currently an editorial board member of 12 professional journals in ethics, bioethics, and health policy, and has lectured widely at national and international conferences, professional societies, universities, and health care institutions. Current research focuses on ethical issues in health resource prioritization, with a special focus on cost-effectiveness analysis, and on genetic selection for enhancement and to prevent disability.

Michael Chernew, Ph.D., is a professor in the Department of Health Care Policy at Harvard Medical School. One major area of his research focuses on assessing the impact of managed care on the health care marketplace, with an emphasis on examining the impact of managed care on health care cost growth and on the use of medical technology. Other research has examined determinants of patient choice of hospital and the impact of health plan performance measures on employee and employer selection of health plans. Dr. Chernew is a member of the Commonwealth Foundation's Commission on a High-Performance Health Care System. In 2000 and 2004, he served on technical advisory panels for the Center for Medicare and Medicaid Services that reviewed the assumptions used by the Medicare actuaries to assess the financial status of the Medicare trust funds. On the panels, Dr. Chernew focused on the methodology used to project trends in long-term health care cost growth. In 1998, he was awarded the John D. Thompson Prize for Young Investigators by the Association of University Programs in Public Health. In 1999, he received the Alice S. Hersh Young Investigator Award from the Association of Health Services Research. Both of these awards recognize overall contributions to the field of health services research. Dr. Chernew is a research associate of the National Bureau of Economic Research and is on the editorial boards of *Health Affairs* and *Medical Care Research and Review.* He is also coeditor of the *American Journal of Managed Care* and senior associate editor of *Health Services Research.* Dr. Chernew received an A.B. from the University of Pennsylvania College of Arts and Sciences, a B.S. from the University of Pennsylvania Wharton School (economics), and a Ph.D. in economics from Stanford University, where his training focused on areas of applied microeconomics and econometrics.

Steven B. Cohen, Ph.D., is Director, Center for Financing, Access, and Cost Trends at the Agency for Healthcare Research and Quality (AHRQ). Dr. Cohen directs a staff of approximately 50 highly trained and skilled economists, statisticians, social scientists, clinicians and support staff conducting intramural and supporting extramural research on behalf of AHRQ. He also directs activities necessary to conduct and support a wide range of studies related to the cost and financing of personal health care services.

Studies include analyses of health care use and expenditures by individuals and families for personal health care services, the sources of payment for health care, the availability and cost of health insurance, and health status, outcomes, and satisfaction. Dr. Cohen also leads AHRQ's administration of surveys and development of large primary data sets, including the Medical Expenditure Panel Survey (MEPS), to support health care policy and behavioral research and analyses. Dr. Cohen has authored over 100 journal articles and publications in the areas of biostatistics, survey research methodology, estimation, survey design, and health services research. He has also served as an Associate Professor in the Department of Health Policy and Management at the Johns Hopkins University and the Department of Health Services Administration at the George Washington University. He received his Ph.D. and M.S. in Biostatistics from the University of North Carolina and his B.A. in Mathematics and History, CUNY. He is also a Fellow of the American Statistical Association.

Patricia M. Danzon, Ph.D., is the Celia Moh Professor at the Wharton School, University of Pennsylvania, where she is a Professor and former Chair of the Health Care Management Department, and Professor of Insurance and Risk Management. She is also Chair of the Health Care Management Department. Professor Danzon received a B.A. First Class, in Politics, Philosophy and Economics, from Oxford University, England, and a Ph.D. in Economics from the University of Chicago. Dr. Danzon's previous positions include Associate Professor at Duke University, Research Economist at the Rand Corporation, and Visiting Professor at the University of Chicago.

Professor Danzon is an internationally recognized expert in the fields of health care, pharmaceuticals, insurance, and liability systems. She is a member of the Institute of Medicine and of the National Academy of Social Insurance. She is also a Research Associate of the National Bureau of Economic Research. Board memberships include the Board of the International Health Economics Association. She has served as a consultant on international health care issues to the World Bank, the European Commission Working Group on Pharmaceuticals, the New Zealand Treasury, the Asian Development Bank, and U.S. Agency for International Development. In the United States her consulting experience includes work for the American Medical Association, the American Hospital Association, the Insurance Services Office, the Institute for Civil Justice, the Alliance of American Insurers, and the Pharmaceutical Manufacturers' Association. Professor

Danzon is an Associate Editor of the *Journal of Health Economics* and the *International Journal of Health Care Finance and Economics*. She was previously an Associate Editor of the *American Economic Review*, the *Journal of Risk and Insurance*, and the *Journal of Biolaw and Business*. She has published widely in scholarly journals on a broad range of subjects related to medical care, pharmaceuticals, insurance, and the economics of law.

Michael Drummond, B.Sc., M.Com., D.Phil., is Professor of Health Economics and former Director of the Centre for Health Economics at the University of York. His particular field of interest is in the economic evaluation of health care treatments and programs. He has undertaken evaluations in a wide range of medical fields including care of the elderly, neonatal intensive care, immunization programs, services for people with AIDS, eye health care, and pharmaceuticals. He is the author of two major textbooks and more than 500 scientific papers, has acted as a consultant to the World Health Organization and was Project Leader of a European Union Project on the Methodology of Economic Appraisal of Health Technology. He has been President of the International Society of Technology Assessment in Health Care, and the International Society for Pharmacoeconomics and Outcomes Research. He is currently a member of the Guidelines Review Panels of the National Institute for Health and Clinical Excellence (NICE) in the United Kingdom, and is a Principal Consultant for i3Innovus.

Robert L. Erwin cofounded the not-for-profit Marti Nelson Cancer Foundation in 1994 with his late wife, Marti Nelson, M.D. This advocacy organization, based in Davis, California, provides free assistance to patients seeking help with clinical trial enrollment or other access to experimental therapies. The organization operates through a network of unpaid, ad hoc volunteers, including scientists, physicians, and people with other relevant expertise. The Foundation's website, www.CancerActionNow.org has become a resource for individuals looking for additional information on a variety of cancer-related topics. During the past few years, the Foundation has broadened its services to include provision of technical information and analysis to other advocacy organizations, and has increased its work on complex or controversial policy issues in drug development, approval, and reimbursement that affect groups of patients as well as individuals. Mr. Erwin is also a member of the board of directors of C3: The Colorectal Cancer Coalition (Alexandria, Virginia), and the NorthBay Healthcare Foundation (Fairfield, California). Mr. Erwin serves as a member of the Data and Safety Monitoring Board for the Cancer and Leukemia Group B. He is a member of the Research Committee of the American Society of Clinical Oncology, and a member of the National Cancer Policy Forum. He served as member of the California Breast Cancer Research Council from 1996 to 1999 and was its Chairman from 1997 to 1999. Mr. Erwin is President of iBioPharma, Inc. (Newark, Delaware), a public biotechnology company developing vaccines for the prevention and treatment of infectious diseases. He is also chairman of Novici Biotech, LLC (Vacaville, California). From 2003 until 2007 he was managing director of Bio-Strategic Directors, LLC, a life science-industry consulting firm focused on intellectual property and strategy. He was chief executive officer of Large Scale Biology Corporation from 1992 to 2003 and served as its chairman until 2006. He was chairman of Icon Genetics AG from 1999 until its acquisition by a subsidiary of Bayer AG in 2006. Mr. Erwin is an inventor on several issued and pending patents. He has B.S. and M.S. degrees in zoology and genetics from Louisiana State University.

Lou Garrison, Ph.D., is Professor and Associate Director in the Pharmaceutical Outcomes Research and Policy Program, Department of Pharmacy, at the University of Washington in Seattle. His recent research focuses on designing and conducting economic and outcomes research evaluations of pharmaceutical, biotechnology, and diagnostic products, and on policy issues related to pricing and reimbursement, regulatory risk-benefit analysis, and pharmacogenetics. Prior to joining UW in 2004, Dr. Garrison was Vice President of Health Economics and Strategic Pricing in Roche Pharmaceuticals for 5 years, working and living in Basel, Switzerland, for the final 2½ years. In 12 years at Roche, he eventually directed a department of over 20 staff members charged with developing and implementing economic and quality-of-life strategies to support global pricing, reimbursement, and market access. Before joining the pharmaceutical industry in 1992, Dr. Garrison was Director of the Project HOPE Center for Health Affairs in Maryland, where he conducted numerous domestic and international health policy projects, including health system reform studies and training in Poland and Jamaica. Dr. Garrison has been a member of ISPOR since 1995, and has served in many capacities, including co-chair of the Real World Data Task Force, participant in leadership retreats, and workgroup leader on the Drug Cost Task Force. He has also served as a member of the ISPOR Institutional Council, PhRMA's Health Outcomes Committee, and the IFPMA's Health Economics Advisory Group. Most recently, he has been an advisor to ISPOR's Latin American expansion. Dr. Garrison earned his Ph.D. in economics at Stanford University in 1981. Over his 28-year career, he has made numerous presentations at professional meetings, and provided pharmacoeconomic training both for those within the pharmaceutical industry and outside, including groups as diverse as payors in South Africa and Brazil. He has authored or coauthored over 75 publications and reports.

Jeffrey C. Lerner, Ph.D., has served since 2001 as President and Chief Executive Officer of ECRI Institute. Prior to this, he held the position of Vice President for Strategic Planning for 17 years. He played the key role in setting the course for ECRI Institute's transition from its origins as a medical device evaluation laboratory to a broader health research organization that assesses clinical procedures and drug therapies in addition to medical devices.

He has conceived of, secured funding for, and implemented numerous programs in technology assessment. For example, he was the first Center Director of ECRI Institute's Evidence-based Practice Center (EPC) under the Agency for Healthcare Research and Quality (AHRQ), and Coordinator of the Technical Expert Panel of the National Guideline Clearinghouse (a project sponsored by AHRQ in cooperation with the American Medical Association and the American Association of Health Plans). He also served as a member of the Medicare Coverage Advisory Committee (MCAC) until 2003 and is currently on the Advisory Board of the U.S. Cochrane Collaboration Center. Dr. Lerner maintains a special interest in assistive technology for the disabled and has served as principal investigator on projects for the U.S. Department of Transportation and the Easter Seals Society. He was the first Director of ECRI Institute's Center for Healthcare Environmental Management, which offers programs worldwide. He developed ECRI Institute's annual technology assessment educational conference. In 1992, the Society for Strategic Healthcare Planning and Management of the Hospital Association of Pennsylvania selected him for the Dorinson Award. Dr. Lerner was a member of the Technical Board of the Milbank Memorial Fund in New York and a member of the United States Pharmacopeial Convention in Rockville, Maryland. He served as Chair for 7 of his 22 years on the Board of Governors of the Philadelphia Health Care Academy, a program for high school students living in poverty areas. He is also on the Executive Board of the Greater Philadelphia Life Sciences Congress; a former President of the Board of the Health Strategy Network, a society of healthcare planners and managers; and an associate editor of the *Journal of Ambulatory Care Management*. He is an Adjunct Senior Fellow of the Leonard Davis Institute of Health Economics of the University of Pennsylvania.

Over the past 27 years, Dr. Lerner made major presentations to government agencies and professional organizations worldwide and has written articles, editorials, and book chapters, such as "The National Patient Library: Evidence-based Information for Consumers," which appeared in the winter 1998 issue of the *International Journal of Technology Assessment in Health Care*. Dr. Lerner authored the *Journal of Legal Medicine*'s book review essay of "Rescuing Science from Politics, Regulation, and the Distortion of Scientific Research," edited by Wendy Wagner and Rena Steinzor. Dr. Lerner received his M.A., M.Phil., and Ph.D. from Columbia University, where he was awarded three University President's Fellowships and other honors. His B.A. is from Antioch College, and his business training is from the Wharton School. He also studied abroad at St. Andrew's University, Scotland.

Mary McCabe, R.N., M.A., is Director of the Cancer Survivorship Program at the Memorial Sloan-Kettering Cancer Center, where she is responsible for developing and implementing centerwide comprehensive programs for adult cancer survivors. She is also a faculty member in the Division of Medical Ethics at the Cornell Weill Medical College. A graduate of Trinity College, Emory University, and Catholic University, Mary McCabe held several positions at the National Cancer Institute before joining the Memorial Sloan-Kettering Cancer Center, including Assistant Director of the Division of Cancer Treatment and Diagnosis, Director of the Office of Clinical Research Promotion, and faculty member of the Department of Bioethics at the National Institutes of Health (NIH). Mary McCabe has served as a member of numerous committees, including Co-Chair of the Clinical Research Networks Working Group at the National Institute of Health, Chair of the Clinical Trials Integration Committee at the National Cancer Institute (NCI), the Scientific Advisory Board, and the Lance Armstrong Foundation, and is a faculty member of the NCI Adolescent and Young Adult Oncology Progress Review Group. She is a member of the Oncology Nursing Society, American Society of Clinical Oncology, American Nurses Association, Women in Cancer Research, and American Society for Bioethics and Humanities. Mary McCabe has published numerous peer-reviewed articles, serves on the editorial boards for *Seminars in Oncology Nursing*, *Oncology*, and *Oncology News International*, and is editor of *Oncology for Nurses*. She has received numerous awards, including the American Cancer Society Merit Award, Oncology Nursing Society Leadership Award, NIH Outstanding Performance Award, NIH Director's Award, and the Outstanding Alumnae Award, Emory University.

Harold L. Moses, M.D., graduated from Berea College in 1958 and then obtained an M.D. degree from Vanderbilt University School of Medicine in 1962. After residency training in pathology at Vanderbilt and postdoctoral research training at the National Institutes of Health, he spent 5 years as a faculty member in pathology at Vanderbilt and 12 years at the Mayo Clinic in Rochester, Minnesota, the last 6 of which were as Chair of the Department of Cell Biology. He returned to Vanderbilt 20 years ago as Professor and Chair of the Department of Cell Biology in the School of Medicine. Fifteen years ago he became the Founding Director of the Vanderbilt Cancer Center with a concurrent appointment as the B.F. Byrd, Jr., Professor of Clinical Oncology. He resigned as Chair of the Department of Cell Biology in 1998 to devote more time to the Cancer Center, now named the E. Bronson Ingram Cancer Center. At the end of 2004, he became Director Emeritus of the Vanderbilt-Ingram Cancer Center and the Hortense B. Ingram Professor of Medical Oncology. Dr. Moses is well known for his work on the transforming growth factor-β family of growth regulatory peptides and has received a number of awards for his research. He has served as president of the American Association for Cancer Research, chair of the NIH Chemical Pathology Study Section, is a member of the Integration Panel for the U.S. Army Breast Cancer Program, is Co-Chair of the Breast Cancer Progress Review Group for the National Cancer Institute and Chair of the National Cancer Institute Cancer Centers review panel. He is currently Past President of the American Association of Cancer Institutes, and a member of the Institute of Medicine of the National Academies. He chairs the National Cancer Policy Forum of the Institute of Medicine.

Peter J. Neumann, Sc.D., is Director of the Center for the Evaluation of Value and Risk in Health at the Institute for Clinical Research and Health Policy Studies at Tufts Medical Center, and Professor of Medicine at Tufts University School of Medicine. Prior to joining Tufts, he was on the faculty of the Harvard School of Public Health for 10 years, most recently as Associate Professor of Policy and Decision Sciences. His research focuses on the role of cost-effectiveness analysis and risk-benefit trade-offs in health care decision making. He has conducted numerous economic evaluations of medical technologies, including evaluations of treatments for Alzheimer's disease. He also directs a project to develop a comprehensive registry of cost-effectiveness analyses in health care. Dr. Neumann has contributed to the literature on the use of willingness to pay and quality-adjusted life-years (QALYs) in valuing health benefits. His other research has focused on the Food and Drug Administration's regulation of health economic information, and the role of clinical and economic evidence in informing public- and private-sector health care decisions, including those made by the Medicare program. He is the author or co-author of over 100 papers in the medical literature, and the author of *Using Cost-Effectiveness Analysis to Improve Health Care* (Oxford University Press, 2005). He is a contributing editor of *Health Affairs* and member of the editorial board of *Value in Health*. Dr. Neumann has served as President of the International Society for Pharmacoeconomics and Outcomes Research (ISPOR) and as a trustee of the Society for Medical Decision Making. He has also held various policy positions in Washington, DC, including Special Assistant to the Administrator at the Health Care Financing Administration. He received his doctorate in health policy and management from Harvard University.

Lee N. Newcomer, M.D., M.H.A., is the Senior Vice President, Oncology for UnitedHealthcare. His unit is responsible for improving the quality and affordability of care for the 111,000 cancer patients covered by United-Healthcare. Prior to rejoining United Health Group (UHG), Dr. Newcomer was a founding executive of Vivius, a consumer-directed venture that allowed consumers to create their own personalized health plans. From 1991 to 2000, Dr. Newcomer held a number of positions at UHG, including Chief Medical Officer. His work there emphasized the development of performance measures and incentives to improve clinical care. Prior to joining UHG, he was Medical Director for CIGNA Health Care of Kansas City. Dr. Newcomer is a board-certified medical oncologist; he practiced medical oncology for 9 years in Tulsa, Oklahoma, and Minneapolis (Park Nicollet Clinic). He is currently the Chairman of Park Nicollet Health Services, an integrated system of over 650 physicians and a 400-bed hospital. The group is nationally recognized for its leadership in quality, safety, and lean processes.

Dr. Newcomer earned a B.A. degree in biology from Nebraska Wesleyan University, an M.D. degree from the University of Nebraska College of Medicine, and an M.S. degree in health administration from the University of Wisconsin at Madison. He completed his internship and residency in internal medicine from the University of Nebraska Hospital, and fellowships in medical oncology and administrative medicine from the Yale University School of Medicine and the University of Wisconsin at Madison, respectively.

Greg Rossi, Ph.D., Senior Director Health Economics and Outcomes Research at Genentech Inc., received his doctorate in Molecular Biology and Protein Chemistry from the University College London (UCL) in 1993. Since then he has worked in the biotechnology industry, predominantly in the clinical development of supportive care and antineoplastic therapies in the oncology and hematology therapeutic areas. Between 1996 and 2007 Dr. Rossi was at Amgen, Inc. From 1996 to 2005 he was involved in the development and registration of a number of oncology supportive care therapies including responsibility for the design and conduct of a number of phase II, P3, and postlicensing clinical trials. In these clinical development roles he was responsible for directly interacting with the EMEA, the FDA, and other regulatory agencies. He has also been responsible for interaction with CMS and private payors in the United States, as well as review and input into EU health technology assessments submissions. Between 2005 and 2007 Dr. Rossi was therapeutic area head, Global Marketing, responsible for co-leading the development and commercialization strategy of Amgen's late-stage therapeutic oncology pipeline of seven molecules in phase II and III clinical development. In this role he was responsible for overseeing the development of evidence strategies designed to meet the requirements for EU and U.S. registration, coverage, and reimbursement. Currently Dr. Rossi leads the Health Economics and Outcomes Research group at Genentech with responsibilities in Oncology, Immunology, and Tissue Growth and Repair therapy areas as well as providing development support for product pricing and patient access initiatives. Dr. Rossi is author over 25 clinical research manuscripts and numerous abstracts.

Daniel J. Sargent, Ph.D., Professor of Biostatistics and Oncology at the Mayo Clinic, is the Group Statistician for the North Central Cancer Treatment Group and the director of Cancer Center Statistics at the Mayo Clinic Comprehensive Cancer Center. In this capacity he oversees a group of approximately 50 statisticians at the Mayo Clinic; the accomplishments of this group have been repeatedly cited as outstanding by external peer review. He received his B.S., M.S., and Ph.D. from the University of Minnesota, and has been at Mayo Clinic since graduating in 1996. He is a member of the U.S. Gastrointestinal Cancer Steering Committee, and co-chaired the

Gastrointestinal Committee for the NCI Common Data Elements Project. Dr. Sargent co-chaired a joint NCI-EORTC committee on methodology for tumor marker studies, was a member of the FDA panel on endpoints for colon cancer clinical trials, and currently sits on the NCI Clinical Trials Advisory Committee, which oversees all cancer clinical trials in the United States. He has extensive peer-review activities as a member and chair of a NCI Study section (Subcommittee H—the first statistician in history to chair that study section), membership on several NCI Special Emphasis Panels, and ad hoc reviewing for funding agencies around the world. Dr. Sargent is a chair or member of over 30 data safety and monitoring committees, including chairing the committee for the NCI-funded American College of Radiology Imaging Network. Dr. Sargent has published papers on innovative designs for phase I, II, and III clinical trials as well as advances in survival analysis, meta-analysis, surrogate endpoints, and designs for validating tumor biomarkers. He is the founder and leader of the Adjuvant Colon Cancer Endpoints (ACCENT) collaborative group, which has assembled the world's largest database of individual patient data from adjuvant colon cancer trials (> 33,000 patients). He has authored over 150 peer-reviewed manuscripts, book chapters, editorials, and letters, including first-author publications in the *New England Journal of Medicine*, *Journal of the National Cancer Institute*, *Journal of Clinical Oncology*, *Cancer*, *Controlled Clinical Trials*, *Biometrics*, *Statistics in Medicine*, and *Seminars in Oncology*.

Deborah Schrag, M.D., M.P.H., is a health services researcher focusing on the study of cancer care delivery in the Department of Medical Oncology at the Dana-Farber Cancer Institute. Dr. Schrag describes the patterns and outcomes of cancer treatment in order to determine how well treatments with efficacy established in the clinical trial setting are translated into practice in nonresearch settings. This involves strategic use of observational and found data sources and application of statistical techniques to evaluate the impact of treatment interventions in nonexperimental settings. Recent work has focused on technology diffusion and efforts to determine what determines how rapidly new treatments are adopted and the factors that drive utilization. Dr. Schrag's current project seeks to evaluate the quality of care delivered to indigent patients with cancer who are insured by the State Medicaid programs in New York and California. By using Medicaid enrollment and claims histories linked to other data sources including hospital discharge abstracts and tumor registry data, the goal is to prioritize areas for improving care delivery to the poor. Ultimately, the goal is to inform design of sustainable systems architecture for ongoing surveillance of the quality of cancer care. An alternate theme of her research involves improving the cancer care experience for patients by enhancing data collection, information systems, documentation standards, and ultimately clinician–patient communication. She pursues these research areas through a series of collaborative projects and works with health services researchers, biostatisticians, epidemiologists, clinical trialists, decision scientists, and economists. Dr. Schrag works with a variety of public and private organizations such as state health departments, AHRQ, ASCO, NCCN, CALGB, and ABIM to develop strategies to evaluate and improve the quality of cancer care. Although most of the research questions she is interested in are relevant across the spectrum of malignant disease, as a practicing gastrointestinal oncologist, Dr. Schrag has greatest expertise in GI tumors and has focused to greatest extent on studying these themes with respect to colorectal cancer.

Thomas J. Smith, M.D., is the Massey Endowed Professor of Palliative Care Research and Esteemed Professor of Medicine at the Virginia Commonwealth University—Massey Cancer Center in Richmond. He shares leadership of the Thomas Palliative Care Program with Patrick Coyne, R.N., M.S.N., and codirects the Cancer Control and Prevention Program of Massey with Cathy Bradley, Ph.D. His interests are access to care and improvements in the quality of care. With colleagues Bruce Hillner and Chris Desch (deceased) the group has published articles in the *New England Journal of Medicine, JAMA, JNCI,* and the *Journal of Clinical Oncology* on cost-effectiveness and rational allocation of resources, the quality of cancer care and ways to improve it, and new models of care. Colleague Bruce Hillner and he did the background reports for the Institute of Medicine/ National Research Council 1999 report *Ensuring Quality Cancer Care,* and subsequently published the evidence for less-than-optimal cancer care and ways to improve it in the *Journal of Clinical Oncology.* Dr. Smith recently chaired the Health Economics Service Policy and Ethics (HESPE) program to choose a center for Canada to develop optimal pan-Canadian cancer prevention, detection, treatment, and control strategies. Dr. Smith received the national Humanism in Medicine Award in 2000, and in 2000 and 2006 was voted the Distinguished Clinician on the VCU-MCV faculty. In June 2008 he received the ASCO Statesman award for continued service in creating national practice guidelines. He is the medical director of the

Thomas Palliative Care Unit that opened May 2000, now designated as the national Palliative Care Leadership Center for Cancer by the Robert Wood Johnson Foundation Center to Advance Palliative Care. In July 2005 it won the American Hospital Association Circle of Life award for being the best palliative care program in the country, in 2006 was voted best university program by the International Association for Hospice and Palliative Care, and in 2007 won the LifeNet Award for Service in organ transplantation. In 2008 the VCU's Rural Cancer Outreach Program won the Hematology/Oncology News International HOPE award for leadership in small clinical programs and the HOPE award for clinical excellence for integration of palliative care into regular cancer care. Dr. Smith has an active practice in medical oncology and palliative/hospice medicine, concentrating on new treatments for breast cancer and symptom control. Current grant funding includes G08 LM009525-01 (PI Smith) Truthful Information about Prognosis and Options for People with Advanced Cancer to make truthful information available over the Internet; R01CA116227-02 (Meier; Smith, site PI) Palliative Care for Hospitalized Cancer Patients, and the Virginia Initiative for Palliative Care.

Ellen L. Stovall, President and CEO of National Coalition for Cancer Survivorship, is a 37-year survivor of three bouts with cancer and has been advocating for more than 30 years to improve cancer care in America. Ms. Stovall is a member of the Institute of Medicine of the National Academies' National Cancer Policy Forum, established in May 2005 to succeed the National Cancer Policy Board (NCPB). The Forum allows government, industry, academic, and survivor advocacy representatives to meet and privately discuss public policy issues that arise in the prevention, control, diagnosis, and treatment of cancer. Prior to the establishment of the Forum, Stovall was vice-chair of the National Cancer Policy Board Committee on Cancer Survivorship. In that capacity, she co-edited the Institute of Medicine's report *From Cancer Patient to Cancer Survivor: Lost in Transition*, which addressed the issues adult cancer survivors face. Ms. Stovall serves as vice-chair of the Robert Wood Johnson Foundation's National Advisory Committee to Promote Excellence in Care at the End of Life, and she is the vice-chair of the Foundation's National Advisory Committee for Pursuing Perfection: Raising the Bar for Health Care Performance. Ms. Stovall currently serves on the Boards of Directors of the National Committee for Quality Assurance (NCQA) and the Leapfrog Group, and she participates on a steering committee of the National Quality Forum (NQF) to establish consensus around cancer care quality measures. She also sits on several advisory panels, working groups, and committees of the National Cancer Institute, American Association for Cancer Research, and the American Society of Clinical Oncology. In 1997, Ms. Stovall founded and served as president of THE MARCH ... Coming Together to Conquer Cancer. Through her leadership, this national public awareness campaign focused both national and regional media attention on the issues of cancer research and quality cancer care for all Americans. Recognizing a need for the voice of cancer survivors to be heard during the national debate over health care reform, the Cancer Leadership Council (CLC) was convened in 1993 under her direction. Ms. Stovall also served a 6-year term on the National Cancer Institute's National Cancer Advisory Board (NCAB), an appointment she received in 1992 from President Clinton. Today, Ms. Stovall is frequently called upon to work with administration and congressional staff on a variety of cancer-related policy issues, most notably access to quality cancer care.

Sean Tunis, M.D., M.Sc., is the Founder and Director of the Center for Medical Technology Policy in San Francisco, where he works with health care decision makers, experts, and stakeholders to improve the value of clinical research on new and existing medical technologies. He consults with a range of domestic and international health care organizations on issues of comparative effectiveness, evidence-based medicine, clinical research, and technology policy. Through September 2005, Dr. Tunis was the Director of the Office of Clinical Standards and Quality and Chief Medical Officer at the Centers for Medicare and Medicaid Services (CMS). In this role, he had lead responsibility for clinical policy and quality for the Medicare and Medicaid programs, which provide health coverage to over 100 million U.S. citizens. Dr. Tunis supervised the development of national coverage policies, quality standards for Medicare and Medicaid providers, quality measurement and public reporting initiatives, and the Quality Improvement Organization program. As Chief Medical Officer, Dr. Tunis served as the senior advisor to the CMS Administrator on clinical and scientific policy. He also co-chaired the CMS Council on Technology and Innovation. Dr. Tunis joined CMS in 2000 as the Director of the Coverage and Analysis Group. Before joining CMS, Dr. Tunis was a senior research scientist with the Technology Assessment Group, where his focus was on the design and implementation of prospective comparative effectiveness trials and clinical registries. Dr. Tunis also served as the Director of the Health Program at the Congressional Office of Technology Assessment and as a health policy advisor to the U.S. Senate Committee on Labor and Human Resources, where he participated in policy development regarding pharmaceutical and device regulation. He received a B.S. degree in Biology and History of Science from the Cornell University School of Agriculture, and a medical degree and masters in Health Services Research from the Stanford University School of Medicine. Dr. Tunis did his residency training at UCLA and the University of Maryland in Emergency Medicine and Internal Medicine. He is board certified in Internal Medicine and holds adjunct faculty positions at Johns Hopkins and Stanford University Schools of Medicine.

Peter A. Ubel, M.D., is Professor of Medicine and Professor of Psychology at the University of Michigan, a primary care physician at the Ann Arbor Veterans Affairs Medical Center, Associate Director of the Michigan Robert Wood Johnson Clinical Scholars Program, and Director of the Center for Behavioral and Decision Sciences in Medicine at the University of Michigan. His research explores controversial issues about the role of values and preferences in health care decision making, from decisions at the bedside to policy decisions. He uses the tools of decision psychology and behavioral economics to explore such topics as informed consent, shared decision making, and health care rationing. Dr. Ubel has won many research awards, including a Presidential Early Career Award for Scientists and Engineers from President Clinton in 2000. In 2008, Dr. Ubel was awarded the role of Robert Wood Johnson Foundation Health Policy Investigator and became a member of the World Economic Forum. He is author of *Pricing Life: Why It Is Time for Health Care Rationing* (MIT Press, 2000), *You're Stronger Than You Think: Tapping the Secrets of Emotionally Resilient People* (McGraw-Hill, 2006), and *Free Market Madness: Why Human Nature is at Odds with Economics—and Why It Matters* (Harvard Business Press, 2009).

Neil S. Wenger, M.D., M.P.H., is Professor of Medicine in the Division of General Internal Medicine at UCLA and a consulting researcher at RAND. He is director of the UCLA Healthcare Ethics Center and is chair of the Ethics Committee at the UCLA Medical Center. He also is director of the NRSA Primary Care Research Fellowship in the UCLA Division of General Internal Medicine and Health Services Research. Dr. Wenger is an active general internist and carries out research in the empirical study of clinical ethics, care of and decision making for the older patient, and quality of health care. He directs the Assessing Care of the Vulnerable Elders project, which has developed a quality-of-care assessment system for vulnerable older persons and interventions to improve care for this group. Other areas of interest include medication adherence, teaching clinical ethics, and measuring the quality of end-of-life care.

Janet Woodcock, M.D., is the Director of the Center for Drug Evaluation and Research. She previously held various positions within the Office of the Commissioner, FDA, as Deputy Commissioner and Chief Medical Officer, she shared responsibility and collaborated with the Commissioner in planning, organizing, directing, staffing, coordinating, controlling, and evaluating the agency's scientific and medical regulatory activities in order to achieve the mission of FDA. She also served as the Deputy Commissioner for Operations and Chief Operating Officer, FDA, where she was responsible for overseeing agency operations and crosscutting regulatory and scientific processes at the FDA. Dr. Woodcock has close interactions with diverse constituencies, including the clinical and scientific communities, members of Congress and the administration, national media, patient and consumer advocacy groups, the international drug regulatory community, the regulated industry, and representatives of federal and state agencies. She frequently appears in or is quoted by the national media and has testified repeatedly before Congress. Dr. Woodcock has led many cross-agency initiatives while at the FDA. She introduced the concept of pharmaceutical risk management in 2000 as a new approach to drug safety. She has led the Pharmaceutical Quality for the 21st Century Initiative since 2002. This effort to modernize pharmaceutical manufacturing and its regulation through the application of modern science and quality management techniques has been highly successful in meeting its objectives. She has spearheaded an initiative on pharmacogenomics that has led to unprecedented agency–industry interactions on pharmacogenomics use in drug development. Over the last 2 years, she has been leading the FDA's Critical Path Initiative, which is designed to improve the scientific basis for medical product development. Dr. Woodcock was director of the Center for Drug Evaluation and Research from 1994 to 2005. During this period, review times for new and generic drugs were cut in half, while the standards for quality, safety, and effectiveness were improved. Dr. Woodcock also oversaw initiatives to automate submission and review of applications and adverse event reports. Now nearing completion, these initiatives will allow the center to make much more drug information publicly available. Under Dr. Woodcock's leadership, CDER's regulatory decision making was made more open and transparent to the public. Changes included publishing CDER's regulatory procedures and policies, developing over 100 technical "guidances" that describe regulatory standards, providing an unprecedented degree of participation of consumer and patient representatives in FDA processes, and creating an extensive center website that includes drug reviews and consumer information. Prior to joining CDER, Dr. Woodcock was director of the Office of Therapeutics Research and Review, Center for Biologics Evaluation and Research (CBER). There she oversaw approval of the first biotechnology-based treatments for multiple sclerosis and cystic fibrosis. She also served as Acting Deputy Director of CBER for several years. Dr. Woodcock has earned numerous FDA awards including six Commissioner's Special Citations. She also received a Presidential Rank Meritorious Executive Award, the Nathan Davis Award from the American Medical Association (1999), the Roger W. Jones Award for Executive Leadership from American University (2000), the Public Health Leadership Award (2004) from the National Organization for Rare Disorders (NORD), the VIDA Award from the National Alliance for Hispanic Health (2005), the Leadership Award in Personalized Medicine from the Personalized Medicine Coalition, three HHS Secretary's Distinguished Service Awards, and the HHS Asian-Pacific Network achievement award (2001). Dr. Woodcock received her M.D. from Northwestern University Medical School in 1977. She received her undergraduate degree from Bucknell University. She has held teaching appointments at Pennsylvania State University and the University of California at San Francisco.